say

goodbye

to

emotional

eating

say

goodbye

to

emotional

eating

Barb Raveling

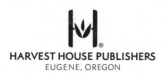

HARVEST HOUSE PUBLISHERS
EUGENE, OREGON

Published in association with the literary agency of WordServe Literary Group, Ltd., www.wordserveliterary.com.

For bulk, special sales, or ministry purchases, please call 1-800-547-8979. Email: Customerservice@hhpbooks.com

Cover design by Faceout Studio, Molly von Borstel

Cover photo © Marish / Shutterstock

Interior design by Angie Renich, Wildwood Digital Publishing

M This logo is a federally registered trademark of the Hawkins Children's LLC. Harvest House Publishers, Inc., is the exclusive licensee of this trademark.

The renewing questions in Part Two first appeared in slightly different form in *I Deserve a Donut (And Other Lies That Make You Eat): A Christian Weight-Loss Resource* and *The Renewing of the Mind Project: Going to God for Help with Your Habits, Goals, and Emotions.*

Say Goodbye to Emotional Eating
Copyright © 2022 by Barb Raveling
Published by Harvest House Publishers
Eugene, Oregon 97408
www.harvesthousepublishers.com

ISBN 978-0-7369-8559-8 (pbk.)
ISBN 978-0-7369-8560-4 (eBook)

Library of Congress Control Number: 2022931414

Printed in the United States of America

22 23 24 25 26 27 28 29 30 / VP / 10 9 8 7 6 5 4 3 2 1

Contents

Part One: Foundations

Part Two: Renewing Exercises

part one

Foundations

Chapter 1

"I Need Ice Cream"

I close my eyes and let out a sigh. *This ice cream is so good,* I think. Spoonful by spoonful, I revel in the joy of it as I devour the whole carton. Then I get up from my perch on the cold concrete at the local grade school and set off for the one-mile walk back to campus.

This was a regular occurrence for me back in my college days in Missoula, Montana. I didn't have a car at the time, so I was forced to walk to my little pig-out sessions. It was inconvenient but necessary. You see, I craved that ice cream. Nothing could stop me from getting it, not even the lack of a car or a cushy place to eat it. I was desperate, and desperate people do whatever they need to do to get their fix.

This type of behavior continued for another 20 years after college. You could tell how my life was going by looking at my body. In the good years I was skinny. In the bad years I wasn't. I was an emotional eater—and emotional eaters gain weight when life is hard.

Most of my pounds were added during the traumas of my life, but a good share of them were added during the celebrations: holidays, vacations, social gatherings—even weekends and evenings were a time for celebration. And what kind of celebration doesn't include food?

My guess is that if we were to sit down for a cup of coffee and a donut, you could tell me a similar story. We both have memories of far too many eating sessions—enough that we've lost hope more than once. For me, eating was that one thing in life that controlled me—the thing I thought I'd never get over. Thankfully, I was wrong.

More than two decades ago, God gave me a discipline that changed my life. First, He used it on my marriage; then He began to use it on my eating habits. That discipline is the renewing of the mind, and it's so effective I've gone 15 years without gaining my weight back.

God can do the same for you. In this book you'll find 100 renewing-of-the-mind exercises designed specifically to help you say goodbye to emotional eating. We'll talk more about how to use those exercises later, but first let's take a look at emotional eating.

Emotional Eating

Emotional eating is letting your *emotions* determine when and what you eat, not your will. So instead of just eating when we're hungry or at mealtimes, we'll eat when we're emotional. When we're happy. When we're sad. When we're annoyed. When we're overwhelmed. You name the emotion—we're ready to eat for it.

Yesterday was a good example. It was 3:00 in the afternoon and I still had a long to-do list that was making me feel discouraged and overwhelmed. I was just thinking how terrible those jobs on the list were, when suddenly I had a brilliant idea. *I'll go to the Dairy Queen for a little blizzard!* I grabbed my car keys and headed for the door, but then I stopped. *No, Barb,* I told myself. *Get up to your office and finish your work.* And surprisingly, I did.

If I had followed through with my little plan, I would have let my emotions—not my will—determine what and when I ate. I call this living by desire, not design. Instead of planning the life I want and following through with it, I'm allowing my emotions and desires to dictate the life I live.

Our culture is all about letting emotions and desires rule, but God isn't. First Corinthians 6:12 tells us, "All things are lawful for me, but not all things are profitable. All things are lawful for me, but I will not be mastered by anything." When I engage in emotional eating, I'm letting my emotions and desires master me. They're telling me *what* to eat and *when* to eat, and I'm sitting back and letting them do that.

But here's the thing: in the old days, I didn't feel like I had any other choice. I would hear Christians—people who never struggled with food a day in their life— tell me, "You have a choice. You can choose to say no to the second bowl of ice cream and the third handful of chips."

But I knew otherwise. That food controlled me hook, line, and sinker, and I was powerless to say no. This made me feel defeated and hopeless. Where was the power of God in my life?

Well, the power of God was in the truth. I'd heard "the truth will make you free" (John 8:32), but I didn't know what that meant at the time. Instead, I just felt like I was doomed to a life of being overweight and waking up each morning with dread, thinking back to everything I'd eaten the night before.

The Truth Will Set You Free

But remember those people who told me I had a choice? They were right. Only the choice was different from what I had originally thought. It wasn't the choice of whether to eat the third cupcake. It was the choice of whether I'd go to the *truth* to be set free from the *desire* to eat the third cupcake.

The truth will make us free—but we usually don't apply that verse to such mundane things as not bingeing on cupcakes when we're feeling emotional. While it's true that the truth sets us free from death to eternal life with God, it's also true that the truth sets us free from the desires that control us.

The more God replaced lies with truth when I went to Him for help with emotional eating, the more I was able to see the beauty of eating with control. Truth changed my desires and allowed me to say goodbye to emotional eating. And when that happened, I was able to lose weight and have kept it off for more than 15 years now.

God can do the same for you no matter how much you have to lose. Because here's the truth: No matter how much extra weight we carry, we all believe the same lies that make us overeat. I've gained hundreds of pounds throughout my life, but I've never been more than 25 pounds overweight. And even at that body size, I dealt with the same lies that I would have dealt with at 100 pounds of extra weight. I experienced feelings of insecurity, shame, despair, and self-condemnation because I wasn't skinny enough.

So part of saying goodbye to emotional eating is taking off the lies that make us overeat. But another part of the journey will be to take off the lies that tell us we have to be skinny to be acceptable, that life is terrible (and no one likes us) if we're not skinny, and that we'll never, ever break free from the control of food.

I hope this book will give you tools you can use to go to God for help with emotional eating and body image. The renewing exercises will help you take charge of your negative emotions and say, "Hey guys, I'm not going to let you be in charge of my life anymore. From now on, I'm living by design, not desire!"

Before we get started, let's look at an overview of the book. In Part One, we'll look at some biblical foundations and practical tips for breaking free from emotional eating. We'll also go over some renewing-of-the-mind techniques that will help you gain victory over emotional eating. In Part Two, we'll put that knowledge to use with 100 exercises you can use in the moment—when everything in you wants to soothe your emotions with food—to walk away, free to wake up in the morning with no regret.

Chapter 2

It's All Good

My husband and kids had gone to bed and the house was quiet. *Finally,* I thought. *My time! I'll just have a little bowl of granola to unwind.* I headed to the pantry and dished myself up a generous bowl of granola.

It was sooo good.

I relished each and every bite as the stress of the day rolled off my shoulders. When I finished, the house was still quiet...and there was still granola in the cupboard. *Why not have another bowl?* I thought. *I've already blown my diet. One more bowl won't hurt!*

Thirty minutes later I'd finished off all the granola and was eating saltine crackers. Not because I love saltines, but because it was the only thing I could find in the pantry that was remotely interesting.

I was eating for emotional reasons. At that stage of my life, I was not a happy camper. My marriage was troubled, my daily chores were mundane, and as an extrovert, I wasn't getting enough adult conversation. And so I ate...and ate...and ate!

I wish I could go back to those days and do things differently. All that eating had an effect on my body—but it was more than the weight gain. My emotional eating was also shaping my character and my relationship with God. You see, God wanted to use those hard days to draw me closer to Him and help me mature. I bypassed His plan for maturity by heading to the pantry for comfort. So instead of getting His perspective on my life as a homeschool mom and an annoyed wife, I was getting instant gratification—deadening the pain with food so I didn't have to grow or mature.

God had allowed the perfect trial in my life to shape and mold me, but He could only do that if I came to Him—not food—for help with the trial.

When we hear the word *trial*, we often think of big things—cancer, death, war, famine. But trials are also little things—noisy days, sinks full of dirty dishes, and not an adult in sight to visit with.

Trials are things that happen to us, but they're also things we don't want to do. As a homeschool mom, teaching my kids to write was a trial for me. Granted, it was a small trial compared to all the other trials in the world, but it was still a big enough trial to lead to emotional eating—and also a big enough trial that it could have led to growth in my character and relationship with God if I would have gone that route.

We can see God's plan for trials in James 1:2-4:

> Consider it all joy, my brethren, when you encounter various trials, knowing that the testing of your faith produces endurance. And let endurance have its perfect result, so that you may be perfect and complete, lacking in nothing.

God wants to use our trials to help us mature. If we endure, we'll grow in our character. We'll grow closer to God. We won't care if we don't get that yummy treat because we'll be lacking in nothing. God will be enough.

We can see how this works on a practical level by looking at my marriage problems back in those young mom days. Let's say my husband, Scott, does something to bug me. I get annoyed and that makes me feel like eating. It looks like this.

1. **Emotion:** Annoyance

2. **Action:** I grab a bowl of ice cream when everyone goes to bed (plus a couple of brownies and a handful of saltine crackers).

3. **Outcome:**
   - Immediate relief: This lasts for five or ten minutes—while I'm eating the ice cream and maybe the first brownie.
   - Immaturity: I don't work through my marriage problems or my own bad habit of being too critical and annoyed all the time.
   - Distance from God: I'm not going to God for help, and my resentment of Scott also interferes with my relationship with God (Ephesians 4:26-27).

- Regret: I wake up the next morning, thinking of what I ate and wishing I hadn't.

- Weight gain: I may not gain weight if I only do this once, but I'll definitely gain if I make a habit of it.

- More negative emotions: Not only do I continue to be annoyed with Scott, but I also experience the negative emotions of despair and hopelessness because I feel like I'll never get over my weight problem.

The interesting thing is that we often think it's the situations themselves that make us overeat. So we might think, *If only my life were easier, I wouldn't overeat.* Here's the truth, though: it's not the situations that make us overeat—it's our habit of using food as a coping mechanism.

If we want to break free from emotional eating, we'll have to develop a new habit of going to God (rather than food) to process our emotions. So in the example we just looked at, if I skip the ice cream (and the brownies and the saltines) after the kids and Scott go to bed and I go to God instead, it will look like this.

1. **Emotion:** Annoyance

2. **Action:** I go to God and renew my mind so I can get rid of the emotion that is causing me to eat, or at least realize that eating isn't a helpful response to that emotion. (We'll talk about what that looks like in the next few chapters and why it makes a difference.)

3. **Outcome:**

   - No immediate relief: Instead, I'm actually looking at my problems— and that's hard. It may involve tears.

   - Intimacy with God: You know how you get close to someone when you go through a hard experience together? It's the same way with God. When you work through a hard problem with Him, you get closer. When I think back on my hard-marriage days, I don't remember how terrible they were. Instead, I remember how sweet that time with God was.

   - Maturity: God taught me how to let go of my critical spirit and stop being so annoyed all the time over little things. That led to enjoying

Scott and others in their as-is condition. This has been life-changing for me.

- The fruit of the Spirit: I experienced peace and joy—and self-control in the area of my eating habits—even though Scott wasn't changing, because I switched my dependence to God rather than Scott to get my emotional needs met.

- No regret: I wake up the next morning, think about what I ate yesterday, and realize with surprise and relief that I actually followed my boundaries!

Was it worth giving up emotional eating for all those benefits? You bet! As God spoke truth to me and met my needs, I learned to become a person who could hold food (and my idea of the perfect life) with open hands. God was giving me the fruit of self-control through walking in the Spirit rather than walking into the pantry (Galatians 5:16, 22-24).

And you know what? God's gifts (maturity and the fruit of the Spirit) were far better than the gifts I was seeking (ice cream and brownies and you name it in the sweets department). I was experiencing firsthand the truth of James 1:17: "Every good thing given and every perfect gift is from above, coming down from the Father of lights, with whom there is no variation or shifting shadow."

The following diagrams illustrate the difference between the two paths we take: going to food or going to God.

Negative emotion → Emotional eating (go to food for help with life) → Growth in physical size, immaturity, and more negative emotions

Negative emotion → Renew our minds (go to God for help with life) → Growth in maturity, the fruit of the Spirit, and intimacy with God

God's gifts are good, but there's just one problem. It's hard to choose God's gifts when you're in an emotional crisis and a yummy treat is either staring you in the face or calling to you from a five-minute drive away.

So what do we do? How can we quell those powerful urges we feel helpless to control? Simple. We renew our minds. Because here's a secret: God's truth changes our desires. We'll see what that looks like in the next chapter.

Chapter 3

The Secret Weight-Loss Weapon

t was a bleak winter day and the kids were bored. "I know," I said, "let's make some chocolate chip cookies!" The kids all cheered and we were off to the kitchen to make some cookies. After all, we needed a little excitement in our lives! It wasn't until years later that I realized I was teaching my kids a lie: *Eating is fun and exciting. It's a great thing to do when you're bored.*

I learned the same lie growing up, and it led to many unwanted pounds. When the kids were little and I was finding the homeschool mom life a little boring, I'd go to our local bakery, buy a slice of gourmet cake, hide it in my dresser drawer along with a fork, and sneak back to my bedroom between chores and classes to have a few bites of cake. Those delightful morsels of yumminess provided me with instant excitement—and a not-so-instant weight gain.

If I wanted to lose weight and keep it off, I had to get the lies out of my system that were driving me back to that dresser drawer. One of those lies was that eating is a great thing to do when you're bored, but I also believed countless other lies. Lies like, *This will make me feel better, I deserve a treat,* and *It's just one bite.* It wasn't until years later that I discovered how to get those lies out of my system. That's when God taught me the importance of renewing my mind.

"Renewing of the mind" can be one of those phrases that goes in one ear and out the other. We've heard it so many times we don't stop to think what it means. Nor do we know how to do it. In fact, it seems like it's something that just happens to us with no effort on our part if we're Christians.

But this isn't true. The renewing of the mind is a spiritual discipline that can help us change those areas of our lives where we feel we'll *never* change—but it *does* require effort. Paul talks about the renewing of the mind in Romans 12:2: "Do not be conformed to this world, but be transformed by the renewing of your mind, so that you may prove what the will of God is, that which is good and acceptable and perfect."

He goes into a little more depth in Ephesians 4:22-24:

> Lay aside the old self, which is being corrupted in accordance with the lusts of deceit, and that you be renewed in the spirit of your mind, and put on the new self, which in the likeness of God has been created in righteousness and holiness of the truth.

Deceit is another word for lie, but it's more subtle. When someone is trying to deceive us, they're not outright lying. Instead, they're telling half-truths that don't really seem like lies. That makes them hard to spot.

We saw this when Jesus was tempted in the desert. If you look at the things Satan said to Jesus, they don't sound like lies. For example, after Jesus fasted for 40 days, Satan asked Him, "Well, if you're the Son of God, why not just turn some stones into bread and then You won't be hungry anymore?" (Matthew 4:3, paraphrased).

It sounded perfectly innocent. It didn't sound like a lie. But Jesus knew what Satan was really saying: *Life is about comfort, Jesus, and You're uncomfortable. Make Yourself comfortable and eat, for goodness' sake!*

Jesus answered and said, "Man shall not live on bread alone, but on every word that proceeds out of the mouth of God" (Matthew 4:4). In other words, *Life isn't about food, Satan; it's about God, and I'm in the middle of a fast right now to help Me prepare for My mission on earth. God will meet My needs, and He is far better at it than food, which just provides a little temporary comfort.*

Jesus answered every one of Satan's temptations with Scripture—and the truth of the Scripture helped Him withstand the temptation. If Jesus had believed Satan's lie that life was about comfort and He deserved a comfortable life, He would have had an intense desire to turn the stones into bread—so intense He would have had a much harder time saying no.

Paul talked about these intense desires in Ephesians 4:22 when he said that lusts—intense desires—actually stem from deceit. We see how that could have worked for Jesus, but we can also see how it works for us.

Remember when I was stashing the gourmet cake in my dresser drawer? Because I believed the lie that the cake would bring me excitement—and that I needed excitement—I felt an intense desire to go to the bakery and get myself a piece of cake.

This led to the old-self behavior of overeating that Paul talked about in Ephesians 4:22-24. I was being corrupted in accordance with the lusts of deceit. Here's what that looked like in diagram form.

Deceit
"I need some excitement in my life to be happy!"

Lust
I felt an intense desire for some exciting cake.

Old-Self Action
I ate the cake.

If I wanted to avoid grabbing the car keys and heading to the bakery, my only hope was to renew my mind like Paul mentioned in Ephesians 4:23. If I had taken the time to renew my mind, I could have taken off the lies that led to the old-man behavior of jumping in the car and put on the truth that would have led to the new-man behavior of saying, "Hey, man doesn't live by excitement alone, but by every word that comes from the mouth of God. I think I'll go to God for help in getting through the day instead of the cake."

It would have looked like this in diagram form.

Truth
"I don't need an exciting life—or treat—to
make me happy. God is enough."

Healthy Desires
I no longer have an intense craving for the cake.

New-Self Action
I stay home and eat with control.

Do you see what would have happened if I'd taken the time to renew my mind before I scurried off to the bakery? My actions would have changed because I'd have seen the truth in black and white. Or as Ephesians 4:24 puts it, I'd be experiencing the righteousness and holiness that comes from the truth.

Truth changes our desires and sets us free (John 8:31-32). It makes us actually *want* to eat with control. I experienced this firsthand when I started renewing my mind about food. It felt like God was taking the blinders off my eyes.

Before renewing, I'd be thinking that the good life was eating what I wanted when I wanted. After renewing, I could see that the good life was eating with control and holding all things—including excitement and cake—with open hands, ready to give them up if necessary. I was experiencing the truth of Romans 12:2: "Do not be conformed to this world, but be transformed by the renewing of your mind, so that you may prove what the will of God is, that which is good and acceptable and perfect."

I was proving that *God's* will—for me to eat with control (Galatians 5:23)—was good, acceptable, and perfect. When previously I had been thinking that *my* will—eating what I wanted when I wanted—was good, acceptable, and perfect.

God transformed me by the renewing of my mind, but it didn't happen in an instant. Instead, I had to keep going back to Him again and again and *again* to renew my mind with truth. When we've lived with lies for so many years—25 years, in my case—it can take a lot of truth to get those lies out of our systems.

Here's why. Every time we've overeaten in the past, we've subconsciously been speaking lies to ourselves. Lies like, *If it's available I should eat it, This is worth it,* and *That first one was so good I should have another one.* We've also told lies about trying to change to ourselves. Lies like, *I'll start tomorrow, I'll never change,* and *I might as well eat since I already broke my boundaries.* We've also told lies about the importance of being skinny. Lies like, *I have to be skinny, People will like me better if I'm skinny,* and *It's terrible to be overweight.*

So we have to renew our minds about the food itself, but we also have to renew our minds about our ability to lose weight and our body image. In this book, I've provided renewing exercises to help you in all three of those areas in addition to renewing exercises to use when you're feeling emotional. Before we get to that, though, let's talk about one more thing we need if we want to break free from the control of food: lifelong boundaries.

Chapter 4

Better with Boundaries

When my sister and I were in high school, we came up with a brilliant new diet. Every three days, we would give up a new food group. Before we gave it up, we'd go out for one last splurge in that particular group.

Now these weren't your main food groups—fruits and veggies, meat and poultry, dairy. No, these were dessert categories—cookies, cakes, ice cream—that sort of thing. So when we went out for our last splurge, we were having some fun treats. We also made sure we had lots of those yummies for the three days prior to giving them up.

The diet was amazing, but it had its faults. The main drawback was that we got so bored with the diet after three weeks (we ran out of treats to give up at that point) that we gave it up. I think it was the only diet I ever gained weight on.

Back in those days I went from one diet to another without batting an eye. This was my (unplanned) eating and weight-loss strategy at the time:

1. Eat what I wanted when I wanted.

2. Gain 10-25 pounds.

3. Go on a million diets.

4. Finally stick to a diet.

5. Lose 2-25 pounds.

6. Repeat the whole process year after year after year.

It never occurred to me to have boundaries *after* reaching my weight-loss goal. That was my chance to live it up! Enjoy life! Eat what I wanted when I wanted!

Unfortunately, eating what I wanted did not lead to weighing what I wanted. Nor did it lead to the lifestyle I wanted—because I absolutely hated going on diets to try to lose all the weight I gained with my live-it-up strategy.

It took me years of renewing my mind to realize that what I really needed was *lifelong* boundaries with food. In other words, I didn't just need boundaries to *lose* weight, but I also needed boundaries to *maintain* my weight. Why? Because I'm a person who, left to her own devices, always eats enough to gain her weight back and then some. Before I go any further, let me explain what I mean by the word *boundaries*.

Boundaries with Food

According to *Merriam-Webster*, a boundary indicates a border or a limit. A playground fence is an example of a boundary. It limits where the kids can play, but that's not all it does. It also cramps their style.

Those little kids would love to run out in the street and look at all those fun, noisy cars—but the fence holds them in and says, "No, kids, you can't play in the street." That doesn't mean the fence is bad. On the contrary, the fence makes their lives better because it protects them from harm.

The same is true for us. Lifelong boundaries in the area of food make our lives better because they keep us safe. Yes, they cramp our style. But you know what? Our style needs to be cramped because there are consequences to eating what we want when we want.

Here are a few of them: Clothes that don't fit. Discomfort. Diabetes. Sore joints. Weight gain. Depression. Heart disease. Hopelessness. Lack of energy. An early death. These are just a few of the enemies that lurk outside the "fence" of our boundaries, waiting to destroy us.

Boundaries also protect us from emotional eating. Remember the definition of emotional eating? It's letting our emotions and desires tell us when and what to eat. This causes a dependence on food and leads to going to food, not God, for help with life. That leads to weight gain, but it also keeps us stuck in a land of immaturity because we're not dealing with our problems.

When we set boundaries, we're making a declaration: "Emotions and desires, we're tired of you guys being in charge! We're taking control back and giving it to the Holy Spirit. From now on, we're going to God—not you—for help with life!"

That's a good thing—not a bad thing. Renewing consistently will help us remember that boundaries are life giving and desirable, not life destroying and to be avoided at all costs. We'll talk about the different types of boundaries in a minute, but first let's take a look at God's purposes for eating.

A Biblical View of Food

Since we know God could have created our bodies any way He wanted, we have to wonder why He designed us to eat on a regular basis. After all, He could have designed us so we never had to eat. That would have saved time and energy as we wouldn't need to grow or prepare food. I thought of three reasons He set it up the way He did.

First, God chose to use food as a means to energize our bodies so we can do the work He calls us to do. The food we eat will either *give* us energy or deplete our energy, depending on what we eat and how much we eat.

Second, God created food to draw us into fellowship. Meals are times for families and friends to gather together and share about their days with each other. We meet with friends for coffee, we have church potlucks, and we have holiday gatherings. Food draws people together and adds to our sense of community.

God also set up meals as a way to fellowship with Him! He set up feast days in the church, and He talks about the banquet we'll share with Him in heaven (Matthew 8:11). When Jesus came to earth, He spent many a meal fellowshipping with both believers and nonbelievers. He also made the effort to have one last special meal with His disciples before He went to the cross, and He told them to do this often in remembrance of Him, instituting the meal we still share as a body of believers (Mark 14:22-25). Eating together was important to Jesus.

Finally, I believe God gave us food to give us pleasure. He didn't create just one type of fruit, grain, or vegetable. Instead, He went out of His way to create a variety of good foods for us to enjoy. Eating is fun. It's a treat to our taste buds and an enjoyable, relaxing experience.

Are Boundaries Bad?

If eating is so fun, why limit it? Because like all God's gifts, eating can get to the point where it controls us—either because we want too much food or because we become obsessed with looking good, which leads to a fixation on food. God doesn't want us to be controlled by food, but to instead use it for the purposes He intended.

This is easy for some people because they grew up with built-in boundaries: they either eat when they're hungry or they only eat at meals. They also eat reasonable amounts of food. They don't eat a whole carton of Ben and Jerry's just because it's good (like I used to do), and they don't eat a bag of potato chips just because they're depressed. Instead, they only think about food when it's time to eat, so it's easy for them to eat with control.

It's not so easy for us because we think about food all the time. Sure, we eat when we're hungry and at meals, but we also eat for other reasons. We eat when we're bored. We eat when we're depressed. We eat when we're stressed. We eat when we're tired. We eat when we see others eating, and we eat when we drive by our favorite bakery and remember how good those white chocolate huckleberry scones are.

If we want to live a life of self-control with food, we'll need to create boundaries that will keep us from thinking about food all the time. In the beginning, those boundaries may make us think about food *all* the time because they're preventing us from our normal pastime—eating what we want when we want! But as we grow into our boundaries and develop a habit of maintaining them, they'll serve their purpose: we'll only think about food when it's time to eat.

And honestly? For me, that's one of the best parts of breaking free from the control of food. Yes, it's nice to look in the closet and see clothes that fit. Yes, it's nice to feel healthy. Yes, it's nice to be able to backpack and climb mountains in my sixties.

But you know what's nicer? Not craving food all the time and not living with a constant feeling of defeat and hopelessness. I hated those days of always thinking about food, always wanting more, never getting enough. Eating things I didn't even like because I'd already eaten all the fun things in the house. I also hated waking up in the morning and remembering the huge quantities I ate the night before and thinking, *I will never get over this.*

The world tells us that more is better and that we'll be happiest when we eat what we want when we want. But I found I was much happier once I developed a habit of following boundaries that *kept* me from eating what I wanted when I wanted. Boundaries help us break free from the control of food, but unfortunately they don't have the power to transform us.

In the old days, I could set boundaries until I was blue in the face, but I couldn't make myself follow them. It was only through hundreds of renewing-the-mind sessions (like the ones you'll find later in this book) that I gained the self-control to actually follow my boundaries.

So as we get into this discussion on boundaries, remember that boundaries are necessary—but they only work if you combine them with consistently renewing your mind until you get to the point where boundaries become a habit. A *habit* is doing something without even thinking about it. That's what we're looking for in the food department—to follow our boundaries without even thinking about it. Let's get deeper into boundaries.

Primary Boundaries

There are two types of boundaries: primary and secondary. Primary boundaries limit how much food we can eat in a day, and secondary boundaries help us follow our primary boundaries. Let's begin with primary boundaries.

Primary boundaries limit the types or quantity of food you can eat by telling you (1) how often you can eat, (2) how much you can eat, or (3) what types of food you can eat. The idea behind number three is that if you limit your food choices, you'll naturally lose weight since they never put things like Dairy Queen blizzards and chocolate cake on the list of foods you can eat in unlimited quantities!

Primary boundaries can either be diet or non-diet boundaries. There are countless diets out there, but only two or three sets of non-diet boundaries: intuitive eating (or variations of intuitive eating such as hunger and fullness), three meals a day (or three meals and a predetermined number of planned snacks), and possibly intermittent fasting.

I put intermittent fasting in the "possible" category because there are so many different ways people do this. Some of the ways include diet-related activity such as calorie counting and a schedule to follow (eating different ways on different days). Others are more non-diet oriented since they don't have as many rules. For example, one popular method is to eat what you want each day during an 8-hour window, and fast for the other 16 hours.

Both diet and non-diet boundaries limit how much you can eat. The following chart shows how some of the most popular primary boundaries limit the quantity of food you can eat in a day.

Primary Boundaries	How Often	How Much	Types of Food You Can Eat
Non-Diets			
Intuitive eating	Only when hungry	Only enough to satisfy your hunger	All foods
Three meals a day*	Only during your meal or snack	A healthy amount with no unplanned second helpings	All foods
Diets			
WW, calories, or carbs	Whenever you want	Only up to a certain number of points, calories, or carbs per day	All foods
Miscellaneous diets: Mediterranean, Trim Healthy Mama, Atkins, keto, etc.	Usually whenever you want, but sometimes these diets will also tell you when to eat	Each program will have its own rules. If they allow you to eat as much as you want, they'll limit the types of food you can eat.	Again, each program will have its own rules, but they'll often limit the types of foods you can eat.

Did you notice that no boundaries allow you to eat what you want when you want? Some programs try to make you think you get to eat what you want when you want—but they don't really allow you to do that. It's helpful to recognize that from the beginning so you don't spend years searching for a program that will help you lose or maintain weight without cramping your style. All food boundaries cramp our style, unfortunately!

As you think about what primary boundaries you want to establish, remember that your current goal may be to lose weight, but your end goal is to develop a habit where food doesn't control you—where you just eat at certain times or under certain conditions without even thinking about it. That doesn't mean you can't choose diet boundaries to lose weight. When I was on WW, I didn't think about food that much because there was only so much I was allowed to eat in a day.

---

* In the United States, intuitive eating seems to be the most popular form of non-diet boundaries, but in many countries, three meals a day is the preferred boundary. France is one of those countries. If they have a snack in France, it tends to be just one and usually around 4:00 p.m. when the kids come home from school. For more, see Jackie McGeown, "How to Snack Like a French Person," *The Local*, August 23, 2019, www.thelocal.fr/guest-blog-how-to-snack-like-a-french-person.

Are Diets Bad?

In recent years, there's been an onslaught of negative press on diets. Let's take a look at some of the criticisms to see if we should throw all diets out the window. Here are four things people say about diets:

1. "Diets lead to obsessing over weight loss."

2. "Diets just make you think about food all the time."

3. "Diets don't work."

4. "Diets aren't God's best for us."

Diets lead to obsessing over weight loss. This criticism of diets puzzled me when I first started writing about weight loss as I don't have an obsessive bone in my body when it comes to diets, exercise, or anything appearance related. Because of that, going on a diet didn't lead to an unhealthy obsession with weight loss or exercise. What I discovered, though, is that not everyone is like me!

In my conversations with intuitive eating weight loss coaches, I discovered that the people they minister to are often highly motivated, Type A people by nature. They're the people who can make a plan and actually follow it. They told me their clients need to learn to listen to their bodies and not just obsessively follow a plan.

People like me, on the other hand, are in the habit of listening to our bodies too much! We do what we feel like doing rather than what our plan tells us to do. So we need to learn to listen to our plan even when we don't feel like it. I lost my weight with WW, and both the points and the weekly weigh-in helped me reign in my tendency to *not* want to follow a plan. I needed that plan and accountability to lose weight!

If you're a person who tends to obsess over counting calories and points, exercising too much, making sure you're eating all the right foods, or just losing weight in general, it may be helpful to consider *not* going on a diet.

Diets are a means of control, and for some people, control is a companion of obsession. Some of the following steps may be helpful if you'd like to escape the obsession:

- Choose non-diet boundaries (see chart on page 28).

- Set limits on how much you can exercise.

- Stop "researching" diets and exercise. In other words, don't click on any links that pop up in your social media feed! You may also want to limit social media in general if looking at the pictures of all those gorgeous, skinny women and studly men make you step into Comparison Land and feel like you have to be as fit as they are.

- Get rid of the scale or limit how often you weigh yourself.

- Spend time renewing your mind about body image. Each time you catch yourself saying things like, "I need to exercise for two hours to make up for all I ate!" or "I'd better just have 500 calories tomorrow since I ate so much today!" or "I can't go to that person's house for dinner because they may not have any healthy choices!" turn to the Body Image section of this book (Part Two) and choose a renewing activity to help you break free from that feeling that you have to be skinny to be acceptable.

It's also helpful to remember than our obsession with skinny doesn't come from the diets themselves. It comes from living in a culture obsessed with skinny. We need to learn to fight against the belief that we have to be skinny (or buff) to be acceptable. That's unbiblical (see Psalm 139:13-14; 1 Samuel 16:7; and 1 Peter 2:9; 3:3-4), but it's also ridiculous.

Life is so much more than what we look like! Just think of who you are as a person: your interests, your hobbies, your giftings, your strengths, the things you love, the way you reach out to people. All those things are far more important than how you look.

And interestingly, the more we accept ourselves in our as-is condition, the easier it will be to follow our boundaries. After all, a lot of those late-night binge sessions can be attributed to beating ourselves up because we broke our boundaries once again and feel like we'll never lose weight.

Diets just make you think about food all the time. I mentioned this briefly early in this chapter, but I think it's important enough to bring it up again in this discussion. The truth is that *any* boundaries will make you think about food all the time in the beginning if you're in the habit of eating without restrictions. Why? Because boundaries make us stop and think, *Wait, I can't eat right now!* And that just makes us want to eat even more because we feel so deprived. So whatever boundaries you choose, anticipate that they'll make you feel like eating all the time in the beginning.

Now if you're a person who tends to obsess over diets and feel like you have to follow them just exactly right and know *exactly* how many points or calories are in a serving, diet boundaries may make you think about food much more often than non-diet boundaries. So again, this is another good reason to strongly consider non-diet boundaries if you're a person who tends to obsess about all things weight loss.

Diets don't work. We've all heard the statistics: 80 to 95 percent of people gain their weight back. These statistics are true, but what's *not* true is that all those people gained their weight back because they lost it on a diet. According to the National Weight Loss Registry—the largest research study of people who've lost at least 30 pounds for at least a year—it doesn't matter how you lost your weight.* It only matters how consistent you are with your boundaries both before and after the diet.

The reason diets have a bad reputation is because we often do one of four things when we diet.

1. We rely on self-control to follow the diet rather than developing a renewing habit. This leads to yo-yo dieting because most people only have enough self-control to follow a diet for one or two weeks.

2. We either choose an unhealthy diet or make a healthy diet unhealthy by saying things like, "I think I'll only have 500 calories instead of 1500 since I'll lose weight faster that way." This leads to starvation mode, which then sends us into binge mode to replace those calories and we end up gaining the weight back.

3. After losing weight on a diet, we go back to eating what we want when we want without switching over to a new set of boundaries. This leads to gaining back what we lost.

4. We develop bad habits on the diet that don't work for us once we switch to non-diet boundaries. For example, we'll get in the habit of eating

---

* "NWCR Facts," The National Weight Control Registry, accessed October 6, 2021, www.nwcr.ws/research. I also emailed the National Weight Loss Registry with this question: "Have you found that one weight loss plan works better than another for losing weight and keeping it off (such as various diets, intuitive eating, intermittent fasting, etc.)?" This was their reply: "The research consistently shows that the specific diet plan has much less of an impact compared to how well a person can stick to it (i.e., adherence). That means it's generally important to select a diet plan that is most compatible with one's preferences and lifestyle. Of course, in order to produce weight loss, the diet plan must be designed to produce an energy (i.e., calorie) deficit."

"free food" or "healthy food" whenever we want, then have a hard time establishing the habit of eating only when we're hungry or only during regular meals and snacks when we switch to non-diet boundaries.

If a diet is going to work, it must be paired with developing good habits, renewing the mind, and going through the work of learning how to switch over to non-diet boundaries when the diet is over, unless we want to follow the maintenance version of the diet boundaries for the rest of our lives (and most people don't!).*

Diets aren't God's best for us. This is by far the hardest portion of this whole book to write because I want to help the people who need to diet without hurting the people who need to *not* diet! If you're a person who obsesses over diets, either skip this section or read it with a mindset of academic interest. This is not a discussion intended to make you think, *Oh, I should go on a diet!* Instead, it's a discussion to give those of you who could be helped by a diet the freedom to choose and embrace a diet.

The questions we need to ask here are these: Does God care what boundaries we use? And are some boundaries more spiritual than others? Unless we see something in the Bible that tells us to eat a certain way, the answer to both of those questions is *no*. In the Old Testament, God gave rules for eating, but He took away those rules in the New Testament.

Remember when Peter had his vision of being able to eat all things in Acts 10? At that time God changed the order of eating. No longer did everyone have to follow certain rules about what types of foods to eat and not eat. In fact, they no longer had to follow any eating rules—because God didn't replace the old rules with new rules. Because of that we can assume that no one set of boundaries is more spiritual than another. God gave us freedom to throw the old food rules out the window and choose our own pathway for eating.

That doesn't mean we can eat with abandon. God still left His principles in place: No gluttony, for example. No making food an idol. No being controlled by food. No making *skinny* an idol. But within the context of those biblical principles, we have freedom.

As you think about choosing between diet or non-diet boundaries, remember

---

* For help transitioning from diet boundaries to maintenance, check out my YouTube video, "How to Transition from Weight Loss to Maintenance."

that there are advantages and disadvantages to both. The advantage of using a diet to lose your weight is that if you follow the diet exactly, you will lose your weight. If you try losing your weight with intuitive eating, three meals a day, or intermittent fasting, there's a bit of a learning curve.* You'll have to play with it to see how much to eat within those guidelines and still lose weight.

The disadvantage of using a diet to lose your weight—besides the fact that you may have to do things like measure and weigh your food—is that you'll have to learn a whole new boundary system (intuitive eating, three meals a day, or intermittent fasting) once you lose your weight, unless you choose to follow that diet all your life and just increase your food to a maintenance level.

One of the most common problems I see with women who gain their weight back is that they drop their diet boundaries and only retain one aspect of them, such as "I'll try to eat fewer carbs" or "I'll have more zero-point foods." That's a recipe for weight gain because there are no longer any primary boundaries. It's essential to switch over to a set of non-diet primary boundaries after you lose weight if you choose not to follow the maintenance plan of that particular diet.

If you find yourself engaging in yo-yo dieting—starting and stopping diets all the time—do one of the renewing exercises in this book every time you break your boundaries. That will help you avert the start-and-stop process. You may also want to consider switching to non-diet boundaries and focus on control with eating rather than weight loss. Just remember that you'll still need to renew regularly, since it's just as easy to say, "I'll start tomorrow!" with non-diet boundaries as it is with diet boundaries.

I'll give you some questions in a minute to help you think through the process of choosing primary boundaries, but first let's take a look at secondary boundaries.

Secondary Boundaries

If boundaries were a movie, primary boundaries would be the main actor and secondary boundaries would be the supporting actors. Primary boundaries tell you how much you can eat in a day, and secondary boundaries help you follow through on your commitment.

---

* You'll be able to find help from several sources on how to lose weight with intuitive eating and intermittent fasting boundaries, but there is not a lot out there on how to lose weight with three meals a day. For info on that, check out my YouTube video: "How to Lose (or Maintain) Weight on 3 Meals a Day."

Here's an example. Let's say I'm using intuitive eating boundaries but I always eat too much ice cream. So much that I can't seem to lose weight and I'm getting discouraged. If that were the case, I could make a secondary boundary for ice cream. Following are some examples of different secondary boundaries I might make around ice cream:

1. No ice cream, period.

2. One ice cream cone every time I go on vacation.

3. Ice cream only on Sundays.

4. Only homemade ice cream that I make myself.

Do you see how any of those boundaries would help me cut down on my ice cream consumption? Choose the secondary boundary that gives you the *best* chance of following your primary boundaries in a way that will help you lose or maintain your weight, depending on your goal.

Some other secondary boundaries you might install would be sweets (or potato chips) only on social occasions, no eating after 7:00 p.m., or not having chocolate peanut butter granola in the house unless your spouse hides it and gets it out only when you want a single bowl (and yes, I have that boundary!).

I would avoid making too many secondary boundaries. You don't want to complicate things. Instead, begin with your primary boundaries and just add secondary boundaries if you find you need it to make it easier to maintain your primary boundaries.

Choosing Boundaries

Are you ready to choose boundaries? As you make this decision, remember that God never said, "Make sure you know exactly what food boundaries I want you to use." This is one of those areas where He gives us freedom to choose. We often put off the decision because we don't really want to limit our food. I did the same thing when I was writing my first book.

Before I wrote *Freedom from Emotional Eating*, I spent a lot of time praying over the decision because I dreaded writing it so much. Unfortunately, God never gave me the assurance that He wanted me to write it. Years later, I realized that I'd wanted His assurance because I felt that if I knew He wanted me to write it, that would guarantee that people would want to read it! I believe God didn't give me that assurance because He wanted me to write out of love for Him and others, not from a guarantee that my efforts would be rewarded.

I think we sometimes do the same thing with weight-loss boundaries. We want to know what God wants because we feel that will make us successful in losing weight. Yet God may just want us to work on following any boundaries out of love for Him and a desire to break free from the control of food, rather than a guarantee of weight loss.

So ask God for wisdom, look at your lifestyle and personality, visit with God about the options, and choose a set of boundaries that will work for you. If you have a hard time choosing boundaries, set a deadline for when you need to choose them by—preferably within a week—so you don't have to live in indecision for long.

Following are some questions you can use to help you decide which boundaries to choose.

1. Do you tend to obsess about weight loss? If so, what boundaries in the past have helped you stop obsessing?

2. Would you rather have the guarantee of weight loss that usually comes with following a diet (if you're able to follow it perfectly), or would you rather have non-diet boundaries so you don't need to learn a whole new boundary system once you lose weight? (There is definitely a learning curve that comes with establishing new boundaries, and you may need to go back to renewing your mind a lot to be able to follow them.)

3. If you'd rather have the same set of boundaries for both losing and maintaining weight, what boundaries could you live with for the rest of your life?

4. Are you willing to go through the hassle of having to measure and record your food, or would you rather have boundaries that don't require that? Also, do you have the time, energy, and willpower to prepare any special foods the diet requires?

5. Which sets of boundaries would give you the best chance of not thinking about food all the time, if any?

6. If you have a spouse, family, or roommate(s), which sets of boundaries would work well with your household's eating habits? Would any boundaries hinder God's purpose of fellowship around meals together?

7. Have you lost a considerable amount of weight before? If so, what boundaries did you use each time you lost weight?

8. Do you lose weight best on your own or with a group? (Note: If you lose best with a group, try to choose a set of boundaries that has a group associated with it or consider starting a weight-loss Bible study at your church or with a friend so you can have some group support.)

9. What boundaries fit into your lifestyle well?

10. What boundaries do you feel like choosing at the gut level? Is there any good reason to not choose those boundaries?

Here are some questions *not* to ask when you're trying to choose your boundaries:

1. Which boundaries will make losing weight fun and easy?
2. Which boundaries will allow me to eat what I want when I want?
3. Which boundaries will guarantee weight-loss success?

Sadly, the answer to all of these questions is "None!" You might be thinking, *I can't believe I'm still struggling with this after all these years*, but here's the truth: it's not surprising you're still struggling.

Think of it this way. You're working on something you're not good at (saying no to food), and you're also working on a habit, which means you can't just check it off your list once you've lost weight and move on to other goals. Instead, you have to keep following boundaries for the rest of your life. That's hard for people like us. After all, we *love* food, we have a tendency to eat for emotional reasons, and we aren't opposed to eating large quantities of food. That's a triple whammy! We can't break free without putting a huge amount of effort into renewing our minds so we can change the way we think.

If I hadn't started renewing every time I felt like breaking my boundaries 16 years ago, I wouldn't be free right now. But here's the truth we need to pound into our heads: It takes a lot of renewing to break free. If you start getting discouraged about the weight-loss process, commit to doing one of the renewing activities in section 2 or 3 every time you feel like breaking your boundaries, as that will help you follow them. If you feel like giving up altogether, do one of the renewing activities in section 5, "I'll Never Lose This Weight." I included a lot of exercises in those sections because I remember how hard it was!

Honestly, if I hadn't seen God change me through the renewing of the mind in other areas of my life first, I wouldn't have had the strength to keep renewing about my weight since there were so many times when I thought, *I will never ever get over this.*

My prayer is that the renewing exercises in this book will help you keep going when everything in you wants to quit. The next few chapters will show you how to get the most out of those exercises. If you'd like to choose your boundaries before you get to those chapters, fill in the section below.

My Boundaries

1. I would rather follow diet/non-diet (circle one) primary boundaries at this stage of my life because:

2. My primary boundaries are:

3. I like these boundaries because:

4. My secondary boundaries are:

5. I feel like I need these secondary boundaries because:

6. Even though I love food and it's hard to follow boundaries, I actually want to develop a habit of following my boundaries because:

Chapter 5

Truth Journaling

With my new, cushy, leather-look-alike journal in my lap, I began to write. It was February 28, 2006, and I had already been truth journaling for six years. I had a lot of truth under my belt, but not enough truth in the area of eating to allow me to be free from the control of food.

Truth journaling is the phrase I use to describe my process of writing down lies in my journal and replacing those lies with truth. I discovered it in the year 2000 when I was going through a difficult stage in my marriage. I decided to try a think-positive project to work on my marriage and immediately bought a journal to start working on it.

The plan was that every time I had a negative thought about my husband, I would record it in my journal with a positive thought right next to it. It wasn't long before I discovered that many of my negative thoughts were actually lies. I started replacing lies with truth and called it truth journaling.

God used truth journaling to revolutionize my feelings toward my husband, but He has also used it in other ways—including helping me break from the control of food. This is the first entry I made in that cushy journal back in 2006:

> **Belief:** If everyone is having a good snack, I should have it too.
>
> **Truth:** This isn't a good enough reason to eat. If everyone is jumping off the bridge, would I do it?

Do you see how short and sweet that was? One lie. One truth. Truth journaling doesn't have to take a long time. That said, many people have a hard time getting started with truth journaling. Not only is it difficult to remember what you were thinking before you broke your boundaries, it can also be hard to come up with a truth for each lie.

This book will solve half of your problems in the truth journal department because I've already recorded many lies for you. Each truth journal exercise in this book will have five lies in it. All you need to do is circle the lies you've told yourself, then write a truth for each lie. Following are eight things to look for when you're writing the truth for each lie

1. Look for biblical and practical truth.
2. Find a truth that counteracts the lie.
3. Add enough truth to change your desires.
4. Replace half-truths with full truths.
5. Be on the lookout for "I should" and "That will be terrible."
6. Be kind to yourself.
7. Be willing to journal the same lie over and over and over again.
8. Don't be a perfectionist.

Let's look at some examples of each of these tips.

Tip 1: Look for biblical and practical truth.

When you record the truth, sometimes a Bible verse will spring to mind. If it does, write it down. Other times, you won't think of a Bible verse, but your truth will be based on everything you've read in the Bible. It will be a biblical principle. And sometimes you won't have any element of the Bible in your truth. It will just be a practical truth.

Don't feel like you always have to come up with a biblical truth. Practical truths are also important, and some lies won't have a corresponding biblical truth. For example, if my belief is "I ate like crazy today," my truth will be a practical truth: "No, I ate x, y, and z today. If I'm careful the rest of the day, I'll still be able to follow my boundaries—or at least not go over by too much." Just remember that you won't ever write a truth that goes against the Bible. Following are some examples of the truths we just talked about:

Lie	Bible-Verse Truth	Biblical-Principle Truth	Practical Truth
I want this brownie so I should have it.	"All things are lawful for me, but not all things are profitable. All things are lawful for me, but I will not be mastered by anything" (1 Corinthians 6:12).	Just because I want something, it doesn't mean I should have it. God wants me to live a life of self-control, not being controlled by my flesh. Boundaries help me live a life of self-control, and my boundaries tell me to eat three meals a day and no snacks. If I want a brownie, I need to wait and have it at dinner.	If I were to give in to my want-tos all the time, I would weigh 700 pounds and not be able to fit through the door! I use self-control in other areas of my life, and I need to use it in this area as well.
I deserve a treat after all that work!	"Whatever things were gain to me, those things I have counted as loss for the sake of Christ" (Philippians 3:7).	Our culture teaches us that we shouldn't have to suffer and that we should always be rewarded for work—but Jesus tells us to serve others and lay down our lives to love others well. He demonstrated this philosophy when He died for us on the cross—and when He arose, He didn't say, "And now I deserve a donut!"	It's okay to reward myself for hard work, but it's not a reward if I regret it later—and I will regret this out-of-the-boundary treat.

If you have a hard time figuring out if something is true, ask, "What would Jesus say if He were standing right in front of me? Would He agree this is true?" For example, let's say your belief is "I'm a hopeless case." Would Jesus look you in the eye and say, "Boy, I'm sad to say it, but I agree with you. I only offer hope to some people and I'm sorry, but you're not on the list, dear. I do love you, though."

I don't think He'd say that! Instead, He might say, "I love you! You're My creation, My work of art! And I will create a clean spirit in you. Come to Me and renew your mind. I'll replace those lies with truth, and the truth will set you free. Trust in Me, not your own efforts, and you will have hope. *Everyone* struggles with weakness and sin—sadly, you're not immune to that. But I will help you overcome this *if* you keep coming to Me again and again for help."

When we ask the question, "What would Jesus say?" we won't always know the answer because He's not sitting across the table from us speaking out-loud words. But we can know His truth based on everything He said in the Bible.

Are you ready to give this a try yourself? Fill in the chart below with a Bible-verse truth, a biblical-principal truth, and a practical truth. After you're through, you can see what I wrote. Just keep in mind there's a good chance we'll have different truths. That's okay; often several truths come to mind.

Lie	Bible-Verse Truth	Biblical-Principle Truth	Practical Truth
It's not a big deal if I break my boundaries.			
Eating what I want will make me happy.			

How did that go? Truth journaling is something that will get easier with practice. It helps to see how others do it. As you look at how I filled out the chart below, just remember that you don't need to come up with a Bible verse, a biblical truth, and a practical truth every time you truth journal. This exercise is just to help you get familiar with the different *types* of truth you could write for each lie. Here's how I would fill out the chart:

Lie	Bible-Verse Truth	Biblical-Principle Truth	Practical Truth
It's not a big deal if I break my boundaries.	"Put on the Lord Jesus Christ, and make no provision for the flesh in regard to its lusts" (Romans 13:14).	While this wouldn't be a big deal for someone who doesn't lust over food, it is a big deal for me because I *do* lust over food. God wants me to have self-control in this area of my life so I need to discipline myself for godliness!	While this wouldn't be a big deal if this were a one-time event, it is a big deal if it's a regular event because every time I break my boundaries, it reinforces the idea that I don't actually have boundaries. And I need boundaries to live a healthy life since I tend to eat with abandon when I don't have boundaries.
Eating what I want will make me happy.	"Beware, and be on your guard against every form of greed; for not even when one has an abundance does his life consist of his possessions" (Luke 12:15).	Walking with the Spirit will make me far happier than eating with abandon because He gives me the fruit of the Spirit, which includes joy.	While an out-of-my-boundaries treat does give me happiness in the moment, long term it leads to depression because the overeating habit enslaves me and takes away my hope.

Tip 2: Find a truth that counteracts the lie.

Often people will write a truth—a good truth—but the truth doesn't counteract the lie. Let me show you what I mean. In the chart below, I've listed a lie, a truth that doesn't fit the lie, and a truth that does fit the lie. See if you can see the difference in the various truths.

Lie	Truth That Doesn't Counteract the Lie	A Specific Truth That Counteracts the Lie
No one loves me (because I'm fat).	That's a lie straight out of the pit of hell.	This isn't true. Mary loves me. Jim loves me. Margaret loves me. Many of the people at church love me. And best of all, God loves me! The Bible doesn't say "God only loves skinny people." He loves me in my as-is condition and the vast majority of people I know also love me in my as-is condition. Most of them couldn't care less if I'm overweight.
It's okay to eat since I'm hungry.*	If I wait a little bit the hunger will go away.	While it may be "okay" to eat (I won't go to jail, for example), it's not beneficial because my boundaries say I can only have three meals a day and it's not mealtime. If I break my boundaries to eat—even though I'm hungry—I'll be more likely to develop a habit of always breaking them. And since I want to live a life of control of food, I will be much better off if I do something to get my mind off food and wait another hour until dinner to eat!

If you look at that chart, these are the questions we need to ask to find the truth that counteracts the lie:

1. Is it really true that no one loves me?
2. Is it really okay to eat if I'm hungry?

Do you see how the truths in the second column didn't answer those questions? They may be good truths or even related truths, but they're not truths that match the original lie. You might ask, "Why is it so important to find a specific truth to fit the lie? Aren't all truths good?" While it's true that all truths are good, we need to address the specific lie if we're going to be changed because that is the lie that's making us break our boundaries.

When Jesus was tempted to eat bread in the desert, He answered the temptation with a specific truth: *Man doesn't live by bread alone* (Matthew 4:4). He didn't say, "That's a lie straight out of the pit of hell" because what He really needed to remember in order to resist Satan's offer of food was that man doesn't live by bread alone.

---

* Note: A person with intuitive eating boundaries would *not* list this statement as a lie, since the criteria for that set of boundaries is eating when one is hungry.

In like manner, if we're believing the first lie in the chart—no one loves us—we need to know that people *do* love us. We can add extra truth after the specific truth that counteracts the lie—in fact, the more truth the better—but we do need to make sure we address the specific lie with specific truth first.

Let's try that now with the following chart. In the first column, I've listed two lies. Complete the chart by recording a specific truth to counteract each lie. If you get stuck, use the questions below to help you come up with a specific truth.

1. Is everyone else really eating? And should I eat just because they're eating?

2. Will I really start tomorrow?

Lie	Truth That Doesn't Counteract the Lie	Specific Truth That Counteracts the Lie
Everyone else is eating so I should too.		
I'll start tomorrow.		

How did that go? Here's an example of what you might write for specific truths.

Lie	Truth That Doesn't Counteract the Lie	Specific Truth That Counteracts the Lie
Everyone else is eating so I should eat.	I can still have fun even if I don't eat. I'll just focus on the people.	While it's true they're all eating, that doesn't mean I should eat. After all, what if they were all doing cocaine? I need to make my eating decisions based on what is best for *my* boundaries, *not* on what everyone else is eating! Also, it's not true that everyone is eating. I see that Deidre and Tanya are just having something to drink. I will follow my boundaries and join with them in not eating since I'm not hungry and my boundaries are hunger/fullness.
I'll start tomorrow.	It would probably be better to start today.	If the past is any indication, I have a 5 percent chance of starting tomorrow and actually following through on that. Instead I will probably eat as much as I can tonight, then either wake up tomorrow, start again, and give up by late afternoon, or just wake up and blow it all off for a week or two. My best chance of breaking free from the control of food is to always at least *try* to follow my boundaries, then renew my mind every time I break them. God can help me change!

It's okay to include extra truth—in fact, you'll notice that I did that in most of the examples above. Just make sure your first priority is a specific truth that counteracts the lie, since it's that particular lie that is making you want to break your boundaries.

Tip 3: Add enough truth to change your desires.

If you find yourself doing the truth journaling exercises in this book and your desires aren't changing by the time you finish writing the truth, it could be that you're not writing enough truth. We can see how this works with the lie "I'll start tomorrow" in the last chart.

Let's say I was journaling that lie and I wrote something like "I don't know if

I'll start tomorrow" for the truth. That's a true statement because we *don't* know for sure if we'll start tomorrow. But the more truth we write down, the more we'll get at the heart of the problem.

For me I would need to know that if I look at my past experience, I only have a 5 percent chance of starting tomorrow and continuing on. That's the truth that would get me to see that I'm basically lying to myself, and if I really want to break free from the control of food, I had better keep persevering today. Following are two more examples of adding enough truth to change your desires.

Belief	Minimal Truth	Enough Truth to Change Desires
Once I eat the lemon bars, they'll be gone and no longer able to tempt me.	True.	This may be true, but it's not a good reason to eat them. The Bible tells us to flee from temptation, not "Give into temptation so it will no longer tempt you!"
I'll never get over this.	God will help me get over this.	This isn't true. The Bible says I am transformed by the renewing of the mind, so if I continue to renew my mind, God will transform me at some point. I need to be super diligent about renewing and trust in the process. Know that God will change me in His time! The problem is that I have *not* been renewing consistently lately. I need to spend some time brainstorming ways to make myself renew or possibly get an accountability partner.

Do you see how the extra truth I wrote down would give me insight into the way I operate? This would be far more likely to change my desires. You may also find that writing the truth will stir a new desire in you. In the last example, a new desire was stirred to make renewing a priority and possibly to get an accountability partner. When this happens, try to take the time to follow through on your new intention.

Now let's see if you can give it a try. I'll include a belief in the left column. Record a minimal truth in the middle column and enough truth to change your desire in the third column.

Belief	Minimal Truth	Enough Truth to Change Desire
I need a little excitement in my life.		
There's so much commotion I can't keep track of my eating plan.		

How did that go? Here's an example of how you could truth journal those beliefs.

Belief	Minimal Truth	Enough Truth to Change Desire
I need a little excitement in my life.	I don't *have* to have excitement. I can get along without it.	Jesus never said, "Make sure you have enough excitement in your life. You need it to be happy!" Instead He instructed us take up our cross and follow Him (Matthew 16:24). It's okay to want life to be exciting and to plan exciting things if they're things God would approve of. But it's not okay to make excitement an idol and say, "I have to have excitement to be happy." Hold excitement with open hands and plan some nonaddictive, healthy forms of excitement to look forward to!
There's so much commotion I can't keep track of my plan.	"I can do all things through Him who strengthens me" (Philippians 4:13).	The truth is that there's so much commotion, I don't *want* to keep track of my plan. What I really want to do is emotionally eat to escape the commotion! I will feel so much better, though, if I follow my plan even though there are so many people around. God can help me do this.

If you don't have a lot of time to truth journal, it's okay to write minimal truth. But as often as you can, try to write more truth because that will help change your beliefs. Sometimes you'll feel like God is pouring out truth. When that happens, take some time to talk to God about it and let the truth sink in. I draw little light-bulbs in my journal whenever I learn something through truth journaling that is a new *aha* moment. Taking the time to soak in the truth will help you integrate the truth into your mind and your life.

Tip 4: Replace half-truths with full truths.

Women often tell me they have a hard time telling if what they're believing is a lie or not. This isn't surprising. Often, the lies we believe *look* like truth because we've been saying them for so many years. Here's an example. What if I said something like, "I hate boundaries"? I might just say, "True," and move on to the next belief because I might feel deep down to my core that, yes, I hate boundaries—I want to be able to eat what I want when I want, and boundaries keep me from doing that.

But if I look a little closer, I'll realize that "I hate boundaries" is actually a *half-truth*. While it's true that I hate saying no when I'm presented with a wonderful eating opportunity, it's also true that I actually enjoy some things about boundaries. For example, I enjoy that feeling of being in control. I enjoy waking up in the morning without regrets about what I ate the night before. And I thoroughly enjoy the benefits of following my boundaries: weight loss or maintenance, feeling good, having energy, and more.

So if I were looking for 100 percent truth to counter "I hate boundaries," I wouldn't just write "True." Instead, I would write something like, "While it's true I don't *love* boundaries, it's not true that I hate them. I do enjoy these aspects of boundaries"—and then I would list what I enjoy about boundaries. That would be a full truth.

Here's another example. What if I believed that I'm a hopeless case and I'll never change? While it may be true that things look a little hopeless based on the past years of not being able to lose weight, that doesn't mean I'm a hopeless case. God changes people all the time, and He can change us as well. Not to mention the fact that those past years didn't include enough renewing to change. Life is much more hopeful with regular renewing since God uses that to change us.

It's rare that an all-or-nothing statement is 100 percent true, and the more you catch the half-truths you're believing, the more likely you'll be able to change your attitude and desires.

Tip 5: Be on the lookout for "I should" and "That will be terrible."

Often, we believe something like "This treat is so yummy," but the lie that's really tripping us up is "This is so yummy, *so I should eat it*." Or "I don't know when I'll get this again, *so I should eat it*." Or "Everyone else is eating it, *so I should eat it*."

We do the same thing with worries about the future. We'll say things like, "I'll gain all my weight back," but the lie that's really tripping us up is "I'll gain all my weight back, *and that will be terrible*." Or "I'll be fat for the wedding, *and that will be terrible*." Or "That person will judge me if I fail at yet another weight loss attempt, *and that will be terrible*."

It may not occur to you to put "so I should eat it" or "that would be terrible" down when you're truth journaling, but try to be aware of it and include it when necessary. God can teach us a lot of truth in the so-I-should-eat-it and that-would-be-terrible department!

Following are some examples of tips 4 and 5 in action.

Belief	Truth
I hate exercise.	While it's true I'm not fond of exercise, I don't usually hate it. I just don't feel like doing it. But if I keep doing it every day, one day I will learn to like it. Also, I actually do like some types of exercise such as skiing and hiking.
That pie was so good (so I should have another piece).	I should have another piece of pie if my primary concern is five minutes of fun and excitement and taste sensation. I should also have another piece of pie if I want to gain weight, feel bloated, not fit into my clothes, and regret it later! Since I don't want those last few things, I should not have another piece of pie because it's not worth it for five minutes of fun and excitement!

Are you ready to give this a try for yourself? Write the full truth for each of the lies I've listed.

Belief	Truth
I have no self-control.	
I'll gain my weight back (and that would be terrible).	

Following is what I would write for the truth in this example.

Belief	Truth
I have no self-control.	While I don't have a lot of self-control in this area of my life, I do have a lot of self-control in other areas of my life. I pay off my credit card balance each month. I do the dishes after every meal. I don't do drugs. And even in this area, I don't eat every minute of the day. I do have some self-control! Lord, please help me have more self-control!
I'll gain my weight back (and that would be terrible).	Although I would be very sad if I gained my weight back, it wouldn't be the end of the world. God can help me be content in all situations—even if I gain my weight back. Also, I don't know if I'll gain my weight back. My best chance for not gaining it back will be to renew my mind as much as possible since it is the *truth* that sets me free. Lord, will You please help me renew?

You may have noticed that I added a prayer to the last line of the truth in the second example. I often do that. If you're writing the truth and feel like praying, go ahead and pray. Even though we have some basic guidelines for truth journaling, it's still a freestyle event. The purpose is to replace lies with truth, get a biblical perspective, and grow closer to God, so the more conversations with God you can have while doing it, the better!

Tip 6: Be kind to yourself.

When I was teaching a class on truth journaling, I noticed a disturbing trend. Some of the ladies were using truth journaling to beat themselves up. Here's an example of one of the entries.

> **Beliefs:** Boy, I'm failing big! I'm so disgusted with myself and gluttony! I may as well keep gaining.

> **Truths:** What's going on in me? My head? My heart? Why am I doing this? I don't have to keep eating. Won't solve anything. I can start to write to see if I can get to the bottom of this.

Do you see how the first four sentences of truth are basically saying, "You numbskull! Why are you doing this?" One of the reasons this woman beat herself up is because she was just learning how to truth journal. It would have helped if she had numbered the sentences to look at one lie at a time.

When we don't separate the lies, it's easy to read the whole paragraph and think, *Wow, I am terrible!* When we look at the lies one at a time, we're less likely to go into beat-ourselves-up mode. Following is what this paragraph would look like if she had separated her lies.

Beliefs

1. Boy, I'm failing big!
2. I'm so disgusted with myself and gluttony!
3. I may as well keep gaining.

Truths

1. I am *not* failing big! I'm experiencing *normal* failure as failure is a part of growth. Every single person out there who pursues a big goal also experiences failure along the way. It's inevitable. It's only when I pursue a little goal (such as making a deli sandwich that I've made a million times before) that I don't experience failures along the way. The more I go to God and renew my mind, the better I will get at following my boundaries consistently.

2. This is true, but God does not want me to be disgusted with myself. He wants me to ask forgiveness, accept His forgiveness, and move on. He also wants me to hold *skinny* with open hands—I'll be much less likely to be disgusted with myself if I see myself through His eyes. He doesn't see me as disgusting!

3. No, this is crazy. If I'm doing something I don't like, the sooner I stop, the better! I need to keep renewing my mind and trust God for the results. If I continue to trip up and gain, so be it. This is a stronghold for me so it could happen. But if I renew my mind every time I trip up, I will be filling myself with the truth that will eventually set me free. God is so good, and He will deliver me from this!

As you write truth for the lies in the renewing section of this book, try to be kind to yourself. God, in all His graciousness, does not beat us up. Instead, Romans 2:4 tells us that it is His *kindness* that leads to repentance. If *He* doesn't beat us up, neither should we.

Tip 7: Be willing to journal the same lies over and over again.

The Holy Spirit will bring out different aspects of biblical and practical truth as you truth journal, so don't get discouraged when you find yourself journaling the same lies over and over. That's normal. You may believe the truth this morning right after you truth journal, but there's no guarantee those lies won't be back after lunch.

Usually what happens is you'll truth journal the same lie over and over until one day you hear the truth at the same time you hear the lie. Eventually, you won't hear the lie anymore. Unfortunately, we need to truth journal the same lies count-less times until we start believing the truth on a regular basis.

For example, I have hundreds of truth journal entries in my journals about food, but I almost never truth journal about food anymore—less than five times a year. Why? Because God filled me with so much truth back in the days when I journaled through that issue that the truth still sustains me more than a decade later.

If you decide to truth journal for a specific area of your life, try to have the same attitude you'd have if you were going to college. It will be a lot of work up front, but it will pay off in the end. If you put in the time "studying" to get the truth, you'll eventually live in freedom in that area of your life.

Tip 8: Don't be a perfectionist.

As you look at these different tips, be careful not to let them intimidate you. Some women have told me, "I feel like I have to truth journal just right and this makes me not want to do it." The truth is, there's not a "just right." You could eas-ily write 50 different truths for the same lie. Here's an example. In a coaching class I taught, I asked the women to record a truth for two different lies. As you can see below, each woman wrote a different truth for the same lie, but they were all great truths:

Lie 1: A little cheat won't hurt.

- A little cheat does hurt because it can lead to a big cheat and then starting over again.
- A little cheat always hurts because it causes a cheat snowball and an all-you-can-eat-buffet mindset in me.
- A little cheat is a slippery slope to opening floodgates to binge eating. Small compromises can make way for larger ones.

Lie 2: Food will cure my bad moods.

- Breaking my boundaries will lead to an even worse mood.

- The "cure" is a mirage that disappears in an hour or less. It also creates bad moods for the future!

- Food may temporarily make me feel better, but the truth is that indulging my desires all the time is making me a prisoner.

As you can see, there's no one right way to record the truth to each lie. So just write a truth and don't worry about how it comes out. Truth journaling is something you get better at with practice, so just begin by doing some of the truth journal exercises in this book, and refer back to this chapter if it doesn't seem like the exercises are changing your desires.

Chapter 6

Option Charts

I put my pen down and sighed. I had just finished truth journaling about my husband (back in our hard-marriage days), but I still wasn't completely peaceful. Yes, truth journaling helped me get rid of some lies that were causing me to be annoyed with my husband, but the situation itself hadn't changed. I was still stuck with some unpleasant truths, and I needed the strength to live the way God wanted me to live.

Option charts gave me that strength because they showed me the consequences of my potential actions. For example, if I continued to be critical and demanding with my husband, that wouldn't lead to the marriage I desired. It also wouldn't make me happy or close to God—two other things I desired.

Option charts showed me in a visual way that my best hope for a good marriage, happiness, and a close relationship with God was to do the hard thing—love and accept my husband in his as-is condition. This was my best option since God hadn't given me the power to change my husband.

Option charts showed me the consequences of my actions in marriage, but they can also help us see the consequences of our actions with overeating. When I bite into that smooth, creamy donut with the pink icing on the top, I'm not thinking, *Oh, this treat will lead to weight gain, discouragement, health problems, and hopelessness.* I'm thinking, *This donut will make me sooo happy! Bring on the donut!*

Truth journaling tells me that no, that out-of-the-boundaries donut won't make me happy long-term. But option charts show me how that donut (and a hundred other donuts just like it) will affect my life in other ways. When I fully look at the consequences of my actions, I no longer want the donut.

It's important to look at the consequences of our actions because getting us to ignore consequences turns into one of Satan's best tools. Remember Eve in the garden of Eden? Satan basically said, "Look at how beautiful the forbidden fruit is, Eve! Look at how good it would taste! You're crazy if you don't eat that forbidden fruit. It's not going to kill you. No, you'll just be like God, knowing the difference between good and evil! How could that not be a good thing, Eve?" (Genesis 3:4).

We hear the same little thoughts in our head with the donut. *Look at how good that donut is, Barb! Look at how good it would taste! You're crazy if you don't eat that! After all, when will you ever have the chance to eat something like that again? Grab that donut with gusto! You can start following your boundaries tomorrow!*

If Eve had looked at the consequences of her actions, she would have been far more empowered to say no to Satan. And if I had looked at the consequences of my actions back in the days when I was eating donuts willy-nilly, I would have seen how eating without boundaries was causing havoc in all areas of my life, including my relationship with God because food had become a God-substitute. (And of course Satan loves it when we have God-substitutes.)

In the last chapter we saw how *truth* changes desires, but looking at consequences can also change our desires. For example, if I'm standing on a balcony at the top of a skyscraper in New York City, I won't have the desire to jump because I know the consequence of jumping is to die. If a drug dealer offers me meth, I won't have the desire to buy some because I know the consequence is possible jail time and a life destroyed by drugs.

Likewise, if I look at the consequences of a lifestyle of eating what I want when I want, I'll lose my desire to have an out-of-boundary treat. Option charts help us see the consequences of our actions in the moment—and that will change our desires.

Real-Life Options versus Dream-Life Options

Option charts also help us see what our real-life options are. We need this because, more often than not, we're living in a dream world. For example, we think we can change people who don't want to change if we just think of the right thing to say. We think we'll find that perfect job that we absolutely love where everything is easy and they'll pay us tons of money even though we have no experience. And we think we can find the perfect set of boundaries that will enable us to lose weight without ever having to say no to the things we love.

This isn't reality. It may be reality for people who don't care too much about food or would never dream of eating when they weren't hungry. But for people like you and me—people who love food, who don't mind eating large quantities, and who don't necessarily have an off button when it comes to food—we are going to have to suffer if we want to break free from the control of food. We'll actually have to say no to yummy treats when everything in us wants that yummy treat!

Option charts will give us the strength to say no, just like they gave me the strength to love, accept, and forgive my husband back in the days when I was focused on his faults (and ignoring my own faults) rather than on his many wonderful strengths. Let's see how this works with an eating example.

How to Make an Option Chart

Following is an example of an option chart for eating what you want when you want. The headings at the top show the things we want. The column on the left lists our options. The little arrows show whether that option will get us what we want or not. I'll usually fill in the chart and write my comments, then sit back and look at the chart as a whole. When I see the consequences of uncontrolled eating in black and white, it helps me see that maybe it *is* a good idea to follow my boundaries even when I don't feel like it! Take a minute to look at the chart and then we'll discuss it further.

Options	Closeness to God	Permanent Weight Loss	Peace and Joy
To be able to eat what I want when I want and still lose weight.	**NOT**	**AN**	**OPTION!**
Eat whatever I want with abandon. Don't try to control myself.	↓ No, because I'm turning to food, not God, for help with life.	↓ If I truly followed this policy all the time, I would weigh so much I wouldn't be able to fit through the door.	↑↓ Although I would experience a little joy when I ate the things I wanted, I would also experience a lot of depression since I wouldn't be happy with my weight or health.

Follow my boundaries for a certain amount of time, then eat what I want for the next few days/weeks/months, then go back to following my boundaries for another set period of time.	↓ God doesn't like gluttony, and when I do this, I'm a total glutton during my free-eating periods. He would definitely forgive me, but it would distance me from Him because I wouldn't be going to Him for help. I'd just eat.	↓ No, this is an up-and-down-in-the-weight-department life—a crummy way to live life.	↓ No peace and joy in either situation. I'm either resenting not being able to eat what I want or beating myself up for eating too much. It's feast or famine.
Always try to follow my boundaries but don't worry about following them perfectly. It's okay to fudge a bit in the evenings and on weekends, vacations, and holidays.	↓ Still not relying on God.	↓ No. I still feel like I'm suffering, but I never lose weight. I just maintain—maybe!	↓ It's stressful to always be on a diet and never be successful. I hate living like that—no peace and joy!
Continue trying to be consistent with my boundaries but do it in my own strength (in other words, no renewing or only sporadic renewing).	↓ In a sense, this won't affect my relationship with God. At least it won't make it worse than it is now. But if I do develop a habit of consistent renewing, it could draw me closer to Him.	↓ I've proven over and over that I'm incapable of doing this in my own strength. I need to renew if I want to see permanent weight loss!	↓ No. I either get frustrated because I can't make myself follow my boundaries in my own strength, or I have a run of success with self-control, lose the weight, but then gain it back because I haven't changed the way I think. This does not lead to peace and joy!

Try to follow my boundaries *every* day and renew my mind *every single time* I break or am tempted to break them, in writing.	↑ Renewing brings me closer to God. This is my best chance of being close to Him.	↑ This is my best chance for permanent weight loss.	↑ Yes. Renewing helps me see life from a biblical perspective and remember that God is enough. Shockingly, eating with control (while renewing) is my best chance for peace and joy.

When I do an option chart, I always begin with the option I want to see happen. This is pretty much always an impossible option, just as it is with this chart: I want to be able to eat what I want when I want and still lose weight.

While this might be true for people who don't overeat by nature, it's not true for me. When I eat without boundaries, I *always* gain weight. To drill that truth into my head, I cross out that unrealistic option, and put "NOT AN OPTION!" in huge letters with lots of exclamation points to remind myself that this does not work for me.

The next thing I do is to list my *real-life* options. This isn't a brainstorming session to think of things we can do. It's an evaluation session to see how our current behavior is working for us. Remember Dr. Phil? He always says, "How's that working for you?" Option charts show us how that's working for us.

At the end of the chart, I always list what I call the God option—the option I think He wants me to take. This often feels like the worst option because it's the option that includes dying to myself and saying no to my flesh.

But surprisingly, when I evaluate it, it's actually the best option. Living the way God wants us to live not only enables us to love Him and others well, it also gives us the best life possible because the closer we walk with God—even when it involves sacrifice—the more we experience peace and joy.

Option charts remind me that actions have consequences. Option charts remind me that *overeating* has consequences—and just like with drugs, when I remember that eating outside my boundaries has consequences, I lose my desire to do it.

What I always find when I do option charts—and you can do these for all areas of your life—is that I regularly do those middle options—the ones with all the down arrows. When I see what those options are doing to the rest of my life, it opens up my eyes to how crazy I'm being and I actually *want* to take the option God wants me to take.

Try It Yourself

Are you ready to give this a try on your own? Because option charts are a bit tricky to learn, I'd like you to give it a try with the example I've already given you. I'll provide a blank chart below and you can fill it in with the arrows and explanations. Look back at my example if you get stuck, but try to do it on your own first and then compare it to what I wrote after you've filled out your chart.

I've included eleven option charts in the renewing section of this book and two examples of completed charts in Appendices A and B. Go ahead and try your first option chart now.

Options	Closeness to God	Permanent Weight Loss	Peace and Joy
To be able to eat what I want when I want and still lose weight.	NOT	AN	OPTION!
Eat whatever I want with abandon. Don't try to control myself.			

Follow my boundaries for a certain amount of time and then eat whatever I want for the next few days or weeks or months, then go back to following my boundaries for another set period of time.			
Always try to follow my boundaries but don't worry about following them too perfectly. It's okay to fudge a bit in the evenings and on weekends, vacations, and holidays.			
Continue trying to be consistent with my boundaries but do it in my own strength (in other words, no renewing or only sporadic renewing).			
Try to follow my boundaries *every* day and renew my mind *every single time* I break them, in writing if I can make myself do it (and I will try to make myself do it!).			

How did that go? I hope it changed your desires and made you want to follow your boundaries. Option charts have a learning curve, but they're helpful for changing behavior because they help us see the consequences of our current behavior. Which is often what we need to see to have the desire to change it!

Chapter 7

Scripture Meditations and Renewing Questions

have a terrible time renewing my mind. I just can't seem to make myself do it," my client told me.

"Do you have any idea why that is?" I asked.

"I feel like God is disappointed with me. I've struggled with my weight for so long I feel like He's tired of me coming to Him with the same old problem."

I was on the phone with a coaching client, and I wasn't surprised when I heard her answer. I think most of us have struggled with feeling like God is fed up with us. How can He help being frustrated watching us do the same old things over and over?

If God is frustrated, then He's not the only one. We get frustrated too. We're tired of the same old eating problems year after year after year—and we're also tired of going to God for help with them.

I don't know how many times in my own journey I've pulled out my journal and recorded the same old lies again and the same old truths. The only thing that made it worthwhile at the time was that I knew God loved me and I knew He wanted to help me with my struggle.

So often we think of God as a perfectionist dad, saying, "There is no way I'll love you in that condition. Shape up first and lose some weight for God's sake. *Then* I can love you." Or we think of God as the indifferent dad—not even caring about our lives and looking at us with a ho-hum expression in His eyes as we engage with Him.

God isn't like any of those imaginary people. Instead, God looks at us with love in His eyes and says, "Come here, dear child, and let Me help you." We know He wants to help us because we see what He was like when He came to earth.

Jesus could have died to save us without spending years with the disciples before He went to the cross. Instead, He chose to come as a baby, experience the whole realm of human existence from babyhood to adulthood—and then live several years with His disciples to teach them how to live the Christian life. He *wanted* to walk with them through life and help them, and He also wants to walk through life with us and help *us*.

The Scripture meditations and renewing questions in this book will help you go to God to get that help. When you renew your mind, think of the questions as conversation starters for a visit with a God who loves you and wants to help you break free from the control of food. You may even want to picture Jesus looking at you with love in His eyes and asking you the questions.

Just as with truth journaling, write as much truth as you can when you answer the questions. The more you write down, the more your brain will shift its perspective from cultural to biblical. I've designed the renewing questions to include three types of questions:

1. Questions to help you think about what the Bible says.
2. Questions to help you think about the benefits of doing what the Bible says (or the consequences of not doing it).
3. Questions to help you accept anything you need to accept.

It's important to ask these questions so we can embrace our boundaries rather than just suffering through them and trying to follow them grudgingly. Here's an example. Let's say I have a secondary boundary that says, "No sweets except on social occasions." Imagine that I'm sitting at home and all of a sudden the image of a big, fat cinnamon roll dripping with cream cheese frosting pops into my mind. I could be eating that cinnamon roll in ten minutes if I were to hop in the car and zip over to the Mineshaft Restaurant. The cultural perspective says, "You want a cinnamon roll? Eat it, for goodness' sake! You only live once! Stop with the pesky old boundaries already!"

But the biblical perspective says, *Use self-control. Don't make allowances for the flesh. Walk in a manner worthy of God. Don't let your belly be your God.*

When we see what the Bible says, we have three ways of responding to it: We can ignore it, we can obey grudgingly, or we can embrace God's commands and obey them with a dying to ourselves, sharing in the fellowship of His sufferings. Taking that third option is hard, but it's far better than the second. With the second option, we make the sacrifice but every bone in our body hates it. We feel like we shouldn't have to sacrifice. We feel put upon. We feel like life isn't fair.

The third option is different. It's still a sacrifice—we want the cinnamon roll after all—but we're *embracing* the sacrifice, just like Jesus embraced the sacrifice for us on the cross. The renewing questions will help you embrace the sacrifice of not eating what you want when you want. They'll help you actually *want* to follow your boundaries.

As you answer the Scripture meditations and renewing questions in this book, remember that you're in a conversation with a God who knows how hard it is to die to yourself and live a holy life (Hebrews 4:15-16). He wants to help you. Talk to Him with an open mind, willing to change your attitude. Talk to Him with an open agenda, willing to change your actions. And talk to Him with an open heart, believing that He loves you and leaning on Him for comfort and strength.

Part Two

Renewing Exercises

The next section of this book contains 100 renewing activities. Each of these activities will be a chance for you to take off the lies that make you break boundaries and put on the truth that will make you actually want to follow your boundaries! It's divided into five sections.

1. I'm Afraid to Start: This section will give you a taste of the different types of renewing exercises in this book, in addition to some exercises that were created specifically for when you're ready to begin a new commitment to follow your boundaries. I would begin with these renewing exercises.

2. I Don't Feel Like Following My Boundaries: This section has renewing activities for situations where the food itself is tempting. For example, maybe dinner was so good you want a second helping, or you're going to a gathering where you know they'll have good food, or maybe you just made brownies and you know you'll be tempted to eat too many.

3. I Need Chocolate: This section includes renewing activities for when life isn't going well. These are the times we feel like eating for emotional reasons.

4. I Have to Be Skinny: Use these exercises when you're dissatisfied with your body, you feel like you have to be skinny, or you can't get yourself to exercise.

5. I'll Never Lose This Weight: Often we break our boundaries because we don't just want to break free from the *control* of food—we also want to lose weight—and things aren't going well. Maybe you just broke your boundaries again and want to wait and start tomorrow, or you're tired of the struggle, or you feel like you'll *never* get over this. Use these renewing activities when you feel discouraged about some aspect of weight loss.

As you work through the book, keep the following tips in mind:

- **Try to focus on breaking free from the control of food rather than losing weight.** When you focus on losing weight, it's easy to get discouraged and give up if you find yourself breaking boundaries a lot. But if you focus on breaking free from the control of food, it's not the end of the world if you just broke your boundaries! Instead, every boundary break is an opportunity to renew your mind so you can discover the lies that made you break your boundaries and the truth that will help you *not* break them next time.

- **Trust in the process.** Sometimes when you renew, you'll barely feel like you have enough strength to follow your boundaries. Other times, you may still break your boundaries after renewing. But then there will be times when you feel like God is pouring out truth. If you're not consistently feeling your desires change when you renew in writing, go back to the chapter that discusses that type of renewing activity to see if you can find some tips to make the renewing more effective.

- **Renew in writing as often as possible.** Many women have told me they want to develop a renewing habit, but they hate to write. I understand how they feel because I was that way myself when I first started writing books. I *hated* writing. But here's the thing: it's worth overcoming your hatred for writing and doing hard things so you can experience the good gifts God will bring into your life through the process. You will learn at a much deeper level if you take the time to do the renewing exercises in writing.

  Studies show that the more senses we use, the better the learning. So when you combine reading with writing and then talking to God afterward about what you wrote, you'll get far more out of the renewing exercises in this book. If you absolutely can't force yourself to do these exercises in writing, do them in your head. But it's better to do even a small portion of one exercise in writing than it is to do a whole exercise in your head. Writing will change your desires more deeply than doing the exercises mentally.

- **Renew as soon as possible after breaking your boundaries.** If you do one of the exercises in this book as soon as you break your boundaries, you'll have a far better chance of only breaking them once that day. Here's what that would look like with different boundaries:

  - With intuitive eating boundaries, renew whenever you eat when you're not hungry or whenever you eat more than you need to satisfy your hunger.

- With three-meal-a-day boundaries, renew whenever you have an unplanned snack or second helping. If you're allowing one snack only under certain conditions (such as hunger or social occasions), you'd renew if you had a snack under any other conditions (such as emotional eating or available brownies).

- With calories or WW points, I suggest setting a limit for how many points or calories you can have at each meal, then renewing if you go over the limit. If you say you can have no more than five points for breakfast, renew if you have more than five points for breakfast. This will help you avoid reaching the end of the day with no points or calories left.

- With other diets, renew whenever you break one of its rules. If you're following a plan that doesn't allow you to eat sugar, you'd renew if you ate a donut.

If you can't renew in the moment, renew as soon as possible afterward. That will help you avoid a binge, since we often go into I-might-as-well-eat mode as soon as we break a boundary.

- **Renew twice a day if you're not breaking boundaries.** If you're on a roll and you're *not* breaking any boundaries, it's still important to renew because you're following your boundaries with self-control. One day that self-control will slip, and you'll need the truth at that point. I suggest renewing once in the afternoon and again either right before or after dinner. In my experience, the truth usually lasts for a couple of hours when I renew in writing. So if you renew at 3:00 in the afternoon, you usually won't feel like breaking your boundaries again until dinner, which is why it's helpful to renew again at dinner.

- **Know that you won't need to renew forever about food.** Consistency is the key to long-lasting change. I truth journaled on and off about food for four or five years with little result. It wasn't until I made the commitment to renew *every* time I felt like breaking my boundaries (or after breaking them if I couldn't make myself do it before) that I really started to break free from the control of food. That was 16 years ago, and I've only gone through a couple of small periods (maybe one month each) of having to renew about food since then because the truth from all those truth journal entries has held for all these years, and I've never gained my weight back.

You might be thinking, *But that's so much work!* Fortunately, it doesn't take that much time to renew. Let's say I truth journaled 300 times about food to break free (this is an estimate—I've never counted!). If each truth journal entry took 5 minutes (and that's a generous estimate), that's still only 1,500 minutes, which is 25 hours of time. Would you spend 25 hours to break free from the control of food? I'm guessing you would! Even if each renewing exercise took 15 minutes, that's still only 75 hours.

Consistent renewing in the beginning pays off and you won't need to renew about food forever. If a new trial crops up in your life, you may need to go back to renewing for a season. But overeating will still be a small issue in your life, not a big issue. I was worried about going back to my gain-lose-gain cycle until I remembered that if I broke free from the control of food once with the renewing of the mind, I could always start renewing again if I needed to.

- **Renew about your trials as well as your food.** There are two ways to break free from emotional eating: first, get rid of the negative emotions that make you overeat; and second, learn to say no to overeating even when you're experiencing those emotions. It will be helpful to start working on letting go of negative emotions right away, so I've included renewing exercises in the "I Need Chocolate" section to help you with that. Some of those exercises may take a bit longer because you'll be working through the difficult areas of your life. It can be hard to renew about the things that cause emotional upset (relationships, health concerns, worries about the world, etc.), but it's important to do so because God wants to use our trials to help us mature (James 1:2-4)— not just emotionally, but also in our ability to make practical changes.

- **Work on changing the things in your life that need to be changed.** Emotional eating happens when life is hard. Sometimes those hard things are unavoidable—we can't escape them. But other times, there are things we can do to change life and make it better. As you work on renewing, think of what areas of your life make you eat the most. Is there anything you can do on a practical level to improve those areas?

For example, if a difficult relationship is causing you to turn to food for comfort, you could do the renewing exercise about difficult relationships on page 196 but you could also work on making that relationship better: have that awkward conversation, read a book on relationships, or go to a counselor, for example. If worry about world events is causing you to turn to food for comfort, you could stop watching the news or run for political office and work toward change. If stressing about all you need to get done is causing you to turn to food, you could work on overcoming procrastination, managing your time better, or finding ways to simplify your life.

It's a Process

As you work on saying goodbye to emotional eating, try to remember it's a process. Change usually comes in baby steps rather than by leaps and bounds, and some days it will look like you're walking backward. Each time you make a practical change in some area of your life, you're taking a baby step. And each time you do a renewing exercise in this book, you're taking another baby step.

If you've never renewed before, those baby steps can feel like huge giant leaps! But after a while, you'll grow to love your renewing time because it's a time to connect with God. Try to remember that renewing your mind isn't a task to cross off your list—it's a life vest to grab when you're drowning in a sea of lies. And Jesus is the One holding the life vest.

Use this as a time to fellowship with Him and grow closer to Him as you turn to Him for help with emotional eating and body image. I'm excited to see what God will do in your life as you develop a renewing habit. My prayer is that He will pour out His truth on you and set you free from the control of food.

"I'm Afraid to Start"

Nervous About Trying Again

Truth Journaling

Write truths for the following beliefs.

Beliefs

1. I can't start a new eating plan or people will say, "There she goes again!"
2. It will be too (embarrassing, depressing, discouraging) if I fail.
3. I'm incapable of following a weight-loss plan and losing weight.
4. I'll end up breaking my boundaries, and that will be terrible.
5. Since it's too hard, I shouldn't even try.

Truths

1.

2.

3.

4.

5.

"Do I Really Need Boundaries?"

Advantages-and-Disadvantages Chart

There are many reasons we can't commit to boundaries. One reason is that we want to keep our options open. After all, what if a great eating opportunity crops up and we can't take advantage of it because of our pesky old boundaries?

Another reason we don't choose boundaries is that we're holding out for the *perfect* boundaries that will guarantee success. Never mind that those boundaries don't exist. We feel sure we'll find them if we just keep looking!

Finally, we delay committing to boundaries because we feel we need to know the exact boundaries (for sure) that God wants us to have. Often, what we really want is an assurance that God will help us lose the weight; and we feel if we know what boundaries He wants us to have, that will ensure success.

Renewing our minds will help us see that it's far better to just choose a set of boundaries and get started. One way to renew our minds is with an Advantages-and-Disadvantages Chart. In the chart below, list the advantages and disadvantages of keeping your options open by not committing to boundaries.*

Advantages of Keeping My Options Open (and Not Choosing a Set of Boundaries)	Disadvantages of Keeping My Options Open (and Not Choosing a Set of Boundaries)

---

* If you'd like to see how I filled out this chart, visit BarbRaveling.com/breaking-a-habit-when-you-dont-feel-like-setting-boundaries.

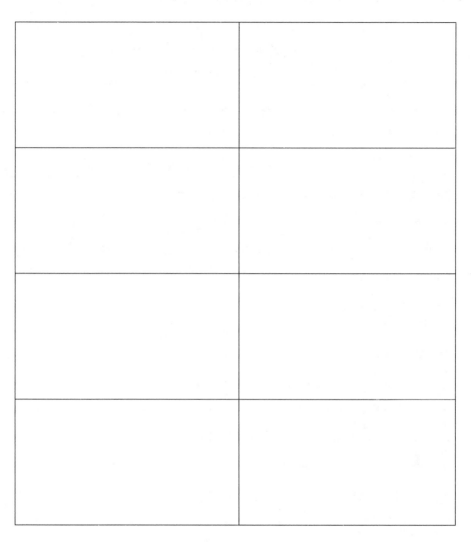

What was your biggest takeaway from filling out this chart?

Would you like to take any action steps based on your takeaway? If so, what are they?

When You Feel Like You Need the Perfect Set of Boundaries

Option Chart

The headings at the top of this chart show the things we want. The rows on the left show our options. Use up and down arrows and comments to evaluate your real-life options so you can see which option would be best.

Options	Consistently Following Boundaries	Closeness to God	Peace and Joy
Find the perfect set of boundaries that will be easy to follow and guarantee weight-loss success.	**NOT**	**AN**	**OPTION!**
Keep searching for the perfect set of boundaries. Don't commit to any boundaries right now since you need to do a little more research.			
Commit to a certain set of boundaries right now but keep second-guessing yourself. Constantly ask, "Should I change to a different set of boundaries?" That way you won't miss any great opportunities.			

Ask God to tell you what boundaries to use, then keep worrying in case you didn't hear God correctly.			
Ask God for wisdom, choose a set of boundaries you think will be helpful, then stick to those boundaries, remembering that it's the renewing of the mind that will change you, not the type of boundaries you choose. (You could give yourself permission to change your boundaries on occasion, but the goal is to stop obsessing about them.)			

Lies About Food You May Have Learned Growing Up

Truth Journaling

If we want to break free from the control of food, we'll need to break free from the lies we learned growing up that make us want to eat more than is good for us. Following are just a sampling of these lies. Circle any lies about food you learned growing up, and record the truth for each lie.

Lies

1. I should be able to eat what I want when I want.

2. Drowning my sorrows in ice cream (or some other great treat) will make me feel better if life isn't going well.

3. There is no need to restrict what I eat unless I'm on a diet.

4. They think I'm dumb for wanting to change my eating habits.

5. There's no reason to try to eat healthy.

6. I won't fit in if I don't eat as much as others do.

7. It's okay to eat as much as I want on holidays.

8. People will think I'm (fill in the blank) if I don't eat what they eat.

Truths

1.

2.

3.

4.

5.

6.

7.

8.

Wonderfully Made
Scripture Meditation

I will give thanks to You, for I am fearfully and wonderfully made;
Wonderful are Your works, and my soul knows it very well.
Psalm 139:14

1. It's easy to get down on ourselves when we're overweight. That's why today's Bible verse is so essential. Do you think this passage applies to everyone, or does it only apply to skinny people? Explain.

2. Why do you think God wanted to make sure you knew that you are awesomely and wonderfully made—so sure that He inspired David to write this verse so it could be included in the Bible He knew you'd read?

3. When you think of your current weight and/or lack of discipline with following your boundaries, what do you feel like doing? (For example, beating yourself up, giving up on your weight-loss plan altogether, or going into crazy exercise or diet mode.)

4. How do you think God would feel about that response? If He wouldn't be excited about it, what do you think He'd rather have you do and why?

5. Spend some time visiting with God about anything that came up in today's meditation, and thank Him for at least five things you love about how He made your body.

"I Don't Want to Renew My Mind"

Option Chart

The headings at the top of this chart show the things we want. The rows on the left show our options. Use up and down arrows and comments to evaluate your real-life options so you can see which option would be best. (Note: You can see how I filled out this chart in Appendix A.)

Options	Peace and Joy	Closeness to God	Consistently Following Boundaries
To be able to lose weight and keep it off without having to renew my mind.	**NOT**	**AN**	**OPTION!** (Romans 12:2)
Give up on renewing and just try to follow my weight-loss plan.			
Renew when it's con-venient, but don't renew when it's not convenient—such as when I'm on a trip or working outside the home.			

Renew once in the morning, but then don't renew again the rest of the day, even if I break my boundaries.			
Renew my mind but don't put my whole effort into it. Just write enough to check it off my list, but not enough to change the way I think.			
Recognize that discipline isn't fun in the moment, but afterward, I will reap joy (Hebrews 12:11). Renew my mind every single time I break my boundaries, even if I'm sick to death of it!			

Challenge: Try to renew two or three times a day (preferably mid-day and late afternoon or evening) for one month and see what benefits you experience.

"I Hate Exercise!"

Truth Journaling

Write truths for the following beliefs.

Beliefs

1. I hate exercise.
2. Exercise is so incredibly boring.
3. I don't want to exercise (so I shouldn't exercise).
4. Exercising isn't that important.
5. I'll just rest for a while now and exercise later.

Truths

1.

2.

3.

4.

5.

"I'll Start Tomorrow"

Renewing Questions

1. What are your boundaries?

2. Is there ever a good or easy time to start following your boundaries?

3. What sacrifices will you have to make to lose or maintain your weight?

4. Will you have to make those sacrifices no matter when you make the commitment to follow your boundaries?

5. What would you gain by starting to follow your boundaries today?

6. What do you think will happen if you don't start today? Be specific.

7. Would it be better to start following your boundaries today, or is there a good reason to wait?

8. Are you the type of person who can go without boundaries in this area of your life and still lose or maintain your weight? Why or why not?

9. Is there anything you need to accept?

10. What will your life and body look like a couple of months down the road if you develop the habit of consistently following your boundaries?

11. When you think of all you have to gain, is it worth following your boundaries today?

When You're Afraid to Start
Scripture Meditation

Do not fear, for I am with you;
Do not anxiously look about you, for I am your God.
I will strengthen you, surely I will help you,
Surely I will uphold you with My righteous right hand.
Isaiah 41:10

When he falls, he will not be hurled headlong,
Because the LORD is the One who holds his hand.
Psalm 37:24

1. What is your biggest fear when you think of trying to lose weight once again?

2. What's the worst thing that can happen if you give it a try even though it's scary?

3. Do you think God wants you to give it a try? Why or why not?

4. According to this passage, why do you not need to be afraid as you begin this journey—or even if you begin it and fail along the way?

5. Spend some time visiting with God about your fears. Soak in His love, take on His strength, and thank Him for all He'll teach you along the way.

"I Don't Feel Like Following My Boundaries"

Eating What You Want When You Want

Scripture Meditation

*Beware, and be on your guard against every form of greed; for not even
when one has an abundance does his life consist of his possessions.*
Luke 12:15

1. What would having an abundance look like when it comes to food?

2. Often, we think we'd be happiest if we could eat as much as we
   wanted without gaining weight. Based on this passage, do you think
   Jesus agrees with us? Why or why not?

3. Jesus isn't trying to be a killjoy. Instead, He knows we won't be happy
   when we start making life about things other than Him. Let's see
   if this is true when we're greedy with food. Think of the life you
   live when you're eating what you want when you want, without
   any boundaries at all. Describe it as fully as possible including your
   emotions, the way your body feels, and how you feel when you wake
   up in the morning remembering what you ate the night before.

4. Now describe a life where you're consistently following your boundaries and consistently renewing your mind so you can remember that life is about God, not food. Describe that life as fully as possible, including your emotions, the way your body feels, and how you feel after you renew your mind and when you wake up in the morning.

5. Which life would you rather live? What is one step you could take today to live that life?

6. Spend some time visiting with Jesus about your current food temptations and ask Him for the strength to follow your boundaries.

Treats in the House

Truth Journaling

Write truths for the following beliefs.

Beliefs

1. This treat is in the house, so I should eat it.
2. After all, it would be so tasty.
3. And I could use a little excitement in my life.
4. One little piece won't hurt.
5. Besides, I deserve a little break today!

Truths

1.

2.

3.

4.

5.

When You're Rebelling Against Your Boundaries

Option Chart

The headings at the top of this chart show the things we want. The rows on the left show our options. Use up and down arrows and comments to evaluate your real-life options so you can see which option would be best.

Options	Consistently Following Boundaries	Peace and Joy	Relationship with God
Eat what I want when I want and still lose or maintain my weight.	NOT	AN	OPTION!
Keep thinking about how it's not fair that I can't eat as much as I want and still lose or maintain my weight.			
Eat in rebellion since it's so unfair that I have to suffer.			

Dwell on how terrible life is when I have to follow my boundaries.			
Be envious and annoyed with everyone who can eat what they want and not gain weight.			
Just break my boundaries for today and then start again tomorrow. I need one day of relaxation!			
Renew my mind as often as necessary to embrace this truth: I am *most* free when I follow my boundaries. Breaking my boundaries keeps me enslaved to my passions.			

Lusting After Food
Scripture Meditation

Put on the Lord Jesus Christ, and make no provision
for the flesh in regard to its lusts.
Romans 13:14

1. What are you lusting after today in the food department?

2. What would you do if you wanted to make provision for the flesh (that is, to make sure the flesh gets as much as it wants to eat)?

3. What will happen if you make provision for the flesh on a regular basis?

4. What would you do if you wanted to set up some safeguards so your flesh *can't* eat as much as it wants to eat?

5. Spend some time visiting with God about your favorite foods. Ask Him to give you wisdom to make helpful boundaries and the strength to follow them.

When You're at a Social Gathering
Truth Journaling

Write truths for the following beliefs.

Beliefs

1. It's a social gathering! I should live it up!
2. I'll never see all this great food again so I should eat as much as possible.
3. Besides, people will think I'm strange if I don't eat.
4. I don't want to make the host unhappy by not eating.
5. Plus everyone else is eating so I should be able to eat.

Truths

1.

2.

3.

4.

5.

Careless Eating

Renewing Questions

1. What do you feel like eating?

2. Will you break a boundary if you eat that? If so, which boundary will break? Is that a good boundary? Why or why not?

3. In the past, have you been able to eat a bite here or there and still maintain discipline in your eating? What usually happens when you get sloppy with your boundaries?

4. In the long run, are you helping or hurting yourself when you break your boundaries—even by a single bite?

5. If you want to have the best life possible, how will you eat today?

Holding Food with Open Hands
Scripture Meditation

Whatever things were gain to me, those things I have counted as loss for the sake of Christ. More than that, I count all things to be loss in view of the surpassing value of knowing Christ Jesus my Lord, for whom I have suffered the loss of all things, and count them but rubbish so that I may gain Christ.

Philippians 3:7-8

1. What's making you want to break your boundaries right now? (For example, is there good food around, are you on vacation, are you stressed?)

2. What are the benefits of breaking your boundaries in this situation?

3. What are the consequences of breaking your boundaries, especially if you make a habit of breaking them in these types of situations?

4. What would it look like to live a life where you hold food with open hands, always remembering that you really only need God to be happy, not those yummy out-of-boundary treats (even though it seems like you need them)?

5. Spend some time thanking God for who He is in your life, letting go of your have-to-haves, and remembering that He is enough.

Eating the Second Piece

Truth Journaling

Write truths for the following beliefs.

Beliefs

1. This is so great.
2. One more will be even better.
3. One piece is not enough.
4. I don't know when I'll get this again.
5. If it's available to eat, I should eat it!

Truths

1.

2.

3.

4.

5.

"My Boundaries Aren't Worth Keeping"
Scripture Meditation

*All things are lawful for me, but not all things are profitable. All
things are lawful for me, but I will not be mastered by anything.*
1 Corinthians 6:12

1. How or what do you feel like eating today? Is it lawful for you to eat
   that way?

2. When a yummy treat is sitting there in front of our face, we
   often think, *This treat is worth breaking my boundaries!* Yet this
   passage encourages us to ask, "Is it really worth it? Will that really
   be profitable?" Think of your current temptation to break your
   boundaries. Will it be profitable to eat this treat? If not, list the
   consequences of choosing that lawful behavior.

3. Will breaking your boundaries lead toward being mastered by food? Explain.

4. What will you gain or profit if you make the choice to follow your boundaries today even though it's hard?

5. Think of the specific temptations you'll face today in the food department. Ask God to give you strength to say *no* to those temptations, and thank Him for what He'll do in your life through following your boundaries.

"I Should Be Able to Eat What They're Eating"
Option Chart

The headings at the top of this chart show the things we want. The rows on the left show our options. Use up and down arrows and comments to evaluate your real-life options so you can see which option would be best.

Options	To Have a Fun and Fair Life	To Be Close to God and/or Experience His Peace and Joy	Consistently Following Boundaries
To eat what everyone else is eating (in the same quantities) and still lose weight!	**NOT**	**AN**	**OPTION!**
Follow my boundaries at home but ignore them in social settings because I should be able to eat what everyone else is eating. After all, life should be fair!			
Try to follow my boundaries but don't think about the benefits of following them. Instead think of the disadvantages and feel super deprived and resentful. Be especially annoyed with skinny people who are eating a lot at the social gathering.			

Tell myself I can't have fun unless I eat too. Then eat what everyone else is eating.			
Use my free will to choose my boundaries, then use my free will to *follow* them even when everyone else is eating. Don't get mad at them because I know this is my choice and no one is forcing me to follow my boundaries. Dwell on the benefits of living a life of boundaries and be thankful that I'm following them!			

Problem Foods

Truth Journaling

Write truths for the following beliefs.

Beliefs

1. This will be so good.
2. It will make me happy.
3. It's so good I should have another.
4. After all, two or three is always better than one.
5. I'll just start following my boundaries tomorrow.

Truths

1.

2.

3.

4.

5.

Holiness and Eating
Scripture Meditation

*As obedient children, do not be conformed to the former lusts
which were yours in your ignorance, but like the Holy One who
called you, be holy yourselves also in all your behavior, because
it is written, "YOU SHALL BE HOLY, FOR I AM HOLY."*
1 Peter 1:14-16

1. What do you think holiness looks like when it comes to eating?

2. What's the downside to being holy with eating?

3. What's the upside to being holy with eating?

4. When you think of the advantages and disadvantages of trying to be holy in the way you eat, which life would you rather live and why?

5. Spend some time visiting with God about how hard it is to be holy and your intentions for the day, asking Him for strength to live the way He wants you to live.

Christmas Treats

Truth Journaling

Write truths for the following beliefs.

Beliefs

1. Sweets are great fun to eat.
2. It's Christmas so I'm bound to eat quite a few Christmas cookies and goodies.
3. Christmas wouldn't be any fun without treats.
4. I'll just start being good after Christmas.
5. That way I can live it up and enjoy the holidays.

Truths

1.

2.

3.

4.

5.

Opportunity Eating
Renewing Questions

1. What do you feel like doing?

2. Why do you think this would be a good opportunity to break your boundaries?

3. Does God think this is a good opportunity? Why or why not?

4. Is this a good opportunity to break your boundaries or a dangerous situation where you'll have to be careful *not* to break your boundaries? Explain.

5. Can you think of anything you can do on a practical level to make it easier to follow your boundaries?

Go ahead and do that if you can, and then pray through the verse below for a little more strengthening.

I can do all things through Him who strengthens me.
Philippians 4:13

"I Need This Treat!"
Scripture Meditation

I have learned to be content in whatever circumstances I am. I know how to get along with humble means, and I also know how to live in prosperity; in any and every circumstance I have learned the secret of being filled and going hungry, both of having abundance and suffering need.
Philippians 4:11-12

1. What do you feel like you need to eat today to be happy?

2. Do you think the apostle Paul would agree that you need to eat that to be happy? Why or why not?

3. Why do you think Jesus wants us to be willing to give up all things to follow Him (Luke 14:33)?

4. Paul said he had to *learn* to be content. It didn't come naturally to him and it doesn't come naturally to us. What would you need to do to learn to be content with following your boundaries today?

5. Can you see any advantages to learning contentment?

6. Ask God for the strength to follow your boundaries today. Thank Him for at least five blessings He's showered you with.

Going Out to Eat
Truth Journaling

Write truths for the following beliefs.

Beliefs

1. I deserve this since I'm going out to eat.
2. I need to eat whatever they serve me.
3. It tastes so good I should have more.
4. There's no way I can follow my boundaries in this situation.
5. I don't want to be the person who's not ordering what everyone else is ordering.

Truths

1.

2.

3.

4.

5.

Indulgence Eating
Renewing Questions

1. Why don't you feel like following your boundaries today?

2. What do you feel like eating?

3. How much would you need to eat before you could honestly say, "That's enough. I don't want any more"? Be specific.

4. At that point would you be (a) more satisfied than you are right now, (b) less satisfied than you are right now, (c) about the same as you are right now, or (d) wishing you could take back the whole eating episode?

5. How often will you follow your boundaries if you only follow them on the days you feel like following them? (Be honest.)

6. What will you gain if you follow your boundaries today, even though it's hard?

7. What will you have to sacrifice or accept to follow your boundaries this time?

8. What truth do you need to remember to be happy about the sacrifice?

A Close Walk with God versus a Close Walk with Food

Scripture Meditation

I am continually with You;
You have taken hold of my right hand.
With Your counsel You will guide me,
And afterward receive me to glory.
Whom have I in heaven but You?
And besides You, I desire nothing on earth.
My flesh and my heart may fail,
But God is the strength of my heart and my portion forever.

Psalm 73:23-26

1. One of the hardest things about breaking free from the control of food is getting to the point where we can hold food with open hands—ready and willing to give it up if it doesn't fit within our boundaries. Why do you think it's so hard for us to reach that point?

2. List everything this psalm says about our relationship with God.

3. Spend some time meditating on the truths you just wrote. How could

those truths help you follow your boundaries even though everything in you wants to break them?

4. What happens when we rely on food, not God, to get our emotional needs met?

5. What would you need to do differently to develop a close walk with God rather than a close walk with food?

6. Spend some time visiting with God about your current temptation and ask Him for strength to follow your boundaries.

"It's Just One Bite!"
Truth Journaling

Write truths for the following beliefs.

Beliefs

1. I'll just have this one little bite.
2. It's so small it can't hurt anything.
3. Besides, it's ridiculous to follow these boundaries so exactly.
4. After all, I don't want to be a legalist!
5. I need to live it up a bit more and stop being such a stick-in-the-mud!

Truths

1.

2.

3.

4.

5.

"I Wish I Were Still on Vacation"
Option Chart

The headings at the top of this chart show the things we want. The rows on the left show our options. Use up and down arrows and comments to evaluate your real-life options so you can see which option would be best.

Options	Peace and Joy	Closeness to God	Consistently Following Boundaries
To still be on vacation	NOT	AN	OPTION!
Think about how boring my regular life is and eat fun things since that is the least I can do now that I am back to my super boring life.			
Work in a frenzy to catch up after vacation and stress eat without thinking about it—after all, I'm too busy to think about boundaries!			
Dwell on the good of regular life, hold excitement with open hands, cultivate thankfulness, and follow my boundaries.			

Developing a Habit of Thankfulness
Scripture Meditation

In everything give thanks; for this is God's will for you in Christ Jesus.
1 Thessalonians 5:18

1. Do you think God wants you to give thanks even when you choose to follow those pesky old boundaries in a situation filled with delightful eating opportunities? Why or why not?

2. What happens when you focus on how deprived you are and how you deserve to eat great things whenever you want?

3. Are you feeling more deprived or thankful right now about food? If deprived, what will happen if you start being thankful about your boundaries over the next 24 hours?

4. List five things you're thankful for when you think of your current boundaries. Be specific.

5. Spend some time praising God for who He is and thanking Him for what He's given you. Be specific in your praise and thanksgiving.

"I Would Be Crazy Not to Eat This!"
Truth Journaling

Write truths for the following beliefs.

Beliefs

1. This food is so good I should have another piece.
2. I want it so I should have it.
3. It's there—I have to eat it!
4. Why would I not eat it if it's there to eat?
5. I would be crazy not to eat it.

Truths

1.

2.

3.

4.

5.

Good Food Eating
Renewing Questions

1. On a scale of 1 to 10, how great do you think this food would taste?

2. How much would you need to eat to be satisfied? (If your answer is, "No amount will satisfy me," turn to the emotional eating questions in section 3.)

3. Can you eat this food without breaking your boundaries?
   No: If not, which boundary will you break? Is that a good boundary? Why?

   Yes: If so, will you be more likely to break your boundaries later if you eat this now? Why or why not?

4. How often will you follow your boundaries if you only follow them on the days you feel like following them? (Be honest.)

5. Do you think God wants you to follow your boundaries? Why or why not?

6. Are boundaries easy to follow or do you usually have to give up something to follow them?

7. What will you have to give up to follow your boundaries this time?

8. What will your life and body look like a couple of months down the road if you develop the habit of consistently following your boundaries?

9. When you think of all you'll gain, is it worth the sacrifice?

Out-of-Bounds Gifts versus God's Gifts
Scripture Meditation

Do not be deceived, my beloved brethren. Every good thing given and every perfect gift is from above, coming down from the Father of lights, with whom there is no variation or shifting shadow.
James 1:16-17

1. What "gifts" (that is, out-of-the-boundaries eating opportunities) do you feel like having right now?

2. Read Galatians 5:22-23. What gifts does the Holy Spirit want to give you today?

3. Choose three of the gifts and share how they would help you follow your boundaries today. Be specific.

4. How are God's gifts different from the "gifts" of out-of-boundary treats?

5. Spend some time thanking God for all the non-food gifts He's given you today, and ask for the gifts you need to follow your boundaries.

Delicious Food

Truth Journaling

Write truths for the following beliefs.

Beliefs

1. There is no way I can follow my boundaries with this food in the house.
2. It's unreasonable to follow my boundaries in this situation.
3. I will just go off my boundaries while it's in the house and start again tomorrow.
4. It will be easier to follow my boundaries tomorrow since I won't have this food in the house.
5. This sounds like a brilliant plan!

Truths

1.

2.

3.

4.

5.

Justification Eating

Renewing Questions

1. What do you feel like eating?

2. What boundary will you break if you eat this?

3. How were you planning to justify it?

4. Is your justification valid? Why or why not?

5. If you want to lose weight and keep it off, will you eventually have to make the sacrifice to follow your boundaries all the time, even when it's hard?

6. Imagine that you start a consistent boundaries habit today and continue it for the next five years. How will you feel five years down the road, and why will you feel that way?

7. What can you be thankful for if you move forward today, following your boundaries even though it's hard?

Being Content with Food
Scripture Meditation

Godliness actually is a means of great gain when accompanied by contentment. For we have brought nothing into the world, so we cannot take anything out of it, either.

1 Timothy 6:6-7

1. Paul tells us that godliness is a means of great gain when accompanied by contentment. How would you define godliness? How would you define contentment?

2. What would godly behavior look like with eating? What would contentment look like with eating?

3. Often we think contentment comes from eating what we want when we want. Because of that, we have a tendency to follow our boundaries grudgingly—the opposite of contentment. What happens when you follow your boundaries grudgingly (without contentment)?

4. What would you gain if you followed your boundaries with contentment and thankfulness?

5. Spend some time visiting with God and thank Him for five specific things you *like* about having boundaries with food. These may be things that boundaries give you if you follow them consistently (such as good health) but they may also be how you feel when you're constantly following your boundaries or how God has provided for you during this process of breaking free from the control of food.

Yummy Food in the House

Truth Journaling

Write truths for the following beliefs.

Beliefs

1. I have treats in the house, so I should eat them.

2. There is no good reason not to eat them.

3. It's crazy not to eat treats if they're available.

4. Besides, they will be so yummy.

5. It's worth breaking my boundaries for those treats.

Truths

1.

2.

3.

4.

5.

"I Feel Like Eating"

Advantages-and-Disadvantages Chart

In the chart below, list the advantages of eating what you want when you want and the disadvantages of eating what you want when you want in this current situation. After looking at both columns, is it worth eating this out-of-your-boundaries treat?

Advantages of Eating What You Want When You Want in This Current Situation	Disadvantages of Eating What You Want When You Want in This Current Situation

1. After looking at both columns, is it worth eating this out-of-your-boundaries treat right now?

2. What will you gain if you don't eat it?

3. What will you have to accept if you don't eat it?

When You're Hungry
Truth Journaling

Write truths for the following beliefs.

Beliefs

1. I'm starving.
2. I don't have enough self-control to think about eating rationally, so I won't think about it.
3. I need my energy for the things I still need to do today.
4. Eating will perk me up.
5. I'll just eat what I want now and have less later.

Truths

1.

2.

3.

4.

5.

Vacation or Holiday Eating
Scripture Meditation

*Whatever you do in word or deed, do everything in the name of
the Lord Jesus, giving thanks through Him to God the Father.*
Colossians 3:17

1. What do you feel like doing in the eating department on this trip or holiday?

2. What do you think is driving that desire?

3. Could you eat as much as you want to eat in the name of the Lord Jesus, giving thanks through Him to God the Father? Why or why not?

4. How could you use thankfulness to safeguard your boundaries during this vacation or holiday?

5. Spend some time visiting with God about the temptations you may experience during this vacation or holiday and how to be victorious in the midst of it.

Celebration Eating
Truth Journaling

Write truths for the following beliefs.

Beliefs

1. This is a special occasion so I should eat what I want.
2. I know I said I wouldn't eat that, but this is a one-time thing.
3. This event or accomplishment deserves a celebration!
4. I will *not* go back to my old habits after I eat this.
5. It is worth breaking my boundaries for this.

Truths

1.

2.

3.

4.

5.

"It's Not That Important to Exercise"
Renewing Questions

1. Why do you feel like it's not a big deal if you don't exercise today?

2. If you decide to take the day off, will you be more inclined to take the day off tomorrow as well? Why or why not?

3. Why do you want to develop an exercise habit?

4. Do you think God wants you to develop an exercise habit? Why or why not? What will you need to sacrifice to do what He wants you to do?

5. Is developing an exercise habit worth the sacrifice? Why or why not?

6. What will happen if you're not willing to make that sacrifice? Do you want that to happen?

7. If you want to develop an exercise habit, will you eventually have to make the sacrifice to exercise even when you don't feel like it? If so, what would be the advantage of exercising today?

8. What can you thank God for?

"I'll Exercise Later"

Renewing Questions

1. Why don't you feel like exercising right now?

2. When we don't feel like working out, it's easy to say, "I'll do it later," and move on with life. If you don't exercise right now, what are the chances you'll do it later on a scale of 1 to 10?

3. When is your best chance to follow through on exercising today?

4. Imagine that you start a consistent exercise habit today and keep it going for five years. How will you feel five years down the road, and why will you feel that way?

5. What's the first thing you need to do if you want to exercise right now? (Put on your tennis shoes, grab a water bottle, change into workout clothes, etc.) Why don't you do that right now and see how it goes from there?

"I Need Chocolate"

Casting Your Cares on God (Not Food)
Scripture Meditation

Humble yourselves under the mighty hand of God, so that He may exalt you
at the proper time, casting all your anxiety on Him, because He cares for you.
1 Peter 5:6-7

1. What are you anxious or upset about right now?

2. According to this passage, why should you cast your cares on God rather than on food in this situation?

3. What will happen if you turn to food in this situation and other situations like this? List as many consequences as possible.

4. According to this passage, what will happen if you turn to God in this situation?

5. Which option is better and why?

6. Ask God for wisdom, comfort, and strength for your current trial, then thank Him for five specific things about who He is in this particular situation or about how He has blessed you in other ways.

"I Deserve This Treat!"
Truth Journaling

Write truths for the following beliefs.

Beliefs

1. I'll just have this one little out-of-boundary treat.
2. I don't care if I'm breaking my boundaries.
3. Life is so bad I deserve it.
4. This will make me feel better.
5. It's one little fun thing I can do in a life of "terrible."

Truths

1.

2.

3.

4.

5.

When You Really, Really Need a Treat

Renewing Questions

1. What's going on in your life today that's making you feel so desperate? Be specific.

2. If life is about "living the good life," is this a terrible situation? Why or why not?

3. If life is about loving God and others, is this a terrible situation? Why or why not?

4. How does God feel about you (or the ones you love) in the midst of this difficult situation?

5. What would He like to do for you (or the ones you love) in this difficult situation? (See Romans 5:3-5 and Psalm 27:5.)

6. How do you think He wants you to handle this crisis?

7. What will you (or your loved ones) gain if you do what He wants you to do?

8. What do you think God wants to teach you (or your loved ones) through this trial?

9. What can you thank Him for?

Things Aren't Going Well
Option Chart

The headings at the top of this chart show the things we want. The rows on the left show our options. Use up and down arrows and comments to evaluate your real-life options so you can see which option would be best.

Options	Happiness	Maturity	Relationship with God
To have everything go well all the time in my life.	**NOT**	**AN**	**OPTION!**
Expect everything to be easy and delightful, then get depressed when it's not—because how can I be happy when life is so hard?			
Dwell on the negative. Think about how terrible my life is—how boring it is, how overworked I am, how nothing ever goes right, and how no one loves me.			
Drown my sorrows in ice cream or some other yummy food because if I can't get a great life, I can at least get a great treat!			

Binge-watch Netflix or read novels nonstop because then at least I can watch other (imaginary) people have great lives and escape my own non-great life.			
Use this situation to learn to be thankful in all situations, then work on changing the things I have the power to change (which isn't other people) and God wants me to change, but with realistic expectations of how long the change process takes.			

Eating to Relax
Truth Journaling

Write truths for the following beliefs.

Beliefs

1. There's so much commotion I can't keep track of my plan.
2. I'll just eat whatever until life settles down.
3. Besides, with all this stress I deserve a little treat.
4. Eating will relax me.
5. I need food to stay awake and get my work done.

Truths

1.

2.

3.

4.

5.

Procrastination Eating
Scripture Meditation

*Whether it is pleasant or unpleasant, we will listen to the voice of
the LORD our God to whom we are sending you, so that it may go
well with us when we listen to the voice of the LORD our God.*
Jeremiah 42:6

1. What's the unpleasant thing you want to avoid doing today?

2. Do you think God wants you to do that unpleasant thing? Why or
why not?

3. What do you feel like doing instead? How will it affect you if you do
that?

4. What benefits will you experience today if you do what God wants you to do rather than what your flesh wants you to do?

5. Spend some time visiting with God and asking Him for strength to do your task today. Ask, "What is the first step?" and begin with the first step.

A Life of Good Works versus a Fun, Exciting, and Easy Life

Scripture Meditation

We are His workmanship, created in Christ Jesus for good works, which God prepared beforehand so that we would walk in them.
Ephesians 2:10

1. According to this verse, we are created for good works. What would a life of good works look like in your current living and work situation? List three or four sentences if possible.

2. I sometimes think I was created for a fun and exciting life rather than for a life of good works. What would it look like to live for the goal of a fun and exciting life in your current living or working situation? Would that make you happy? Explain.

3. Although God wants us to focus life on loving God and others, that doesn't mean we can't make tweaks to life to make it more enjoyable. Think of your current life. Do you feel like you need to add more service opportunities to your life or opportunities for fun? Why do you feel that way?

4. Brainstorm some ideas of things you could add to your life to create more opportunities for service or fun based on what you're currently lacking.

5. Spend some time visiting with God about how He'd like you to spend your day, then ask Him to help you keep Him first and hold exciting food (and an exciting life) with open hands.

When Life Is Boring

Truth Journaling

Write truths for the following beliefs.

Beliefs

1. My life is so incredibly boring.
2. I need a little excitement in my life.
3. This treat would be a great way to get some excitement.
4. After all, it's not a big deal if I break my boundaries.
5. I'll just start following my boundaries tomorrow.

Truths

1.

2.

3.

4.

5.

When You're Anxious

Option Chart

The headings at the top of this chart show the things we want. The rows on the left show our options. Use up and down arrows and comments to evaluate your real-life options so you can see which option would be best.

Options	Things Turning Out the Way I Want	Peace and Joy	Closeness to God
Know for sure that things will turn out the way I want them to turn out.	**NOT**	**AN**	**OPTION!**
Continue to obsess and fret about things and always imagine the worst scenario.			
Try to avoid thinking about things and drown my worries in ice cream, alcohol, Netflix, novels, etc.			

Keep talking about my worries with a loved one and ask them for reassurance that things will turn out okay.			
Try everything I can to control the situation (so things turn out okay), even when it's not a situation I can control.			
Look at the situation from a biblical perspective, put my hope in God (rather than in things turning out the way I want), dwell on the good, be thankful, take any action steps God wants me to take, and accept that my fear may come true.			

"Everything Is Going Wrong!"
Scripture Meditation

Hear my cry, O God;
Give heed to my prayer.
From the end of the earth I call to You when my heart is faint;
Lead me to the rock that is higher than I.
For You have been a refuge for me,
A tower of strength against the enemy.
Let me dwell in Your tent forever;
Let me take refuge in the shelter of Your wings.
Psalm 61:1-4

1. What's going on in your life today to upset you?

2. Where do you feel like going for refuge (or what do you feel like eating)?

3. What will happen if you do that for refuge?

4. When we're upset, it can be hard to go to God for refuge. Instead, everything in us craves escape, and we want to take refuge in comfort food. Yet God is such a better refuge. Take a minute to focus on God and see if you can feel His presence (don't worry if you can't—He's still there). Then tell God your struggles and ask Him to help. Finish by praying through today's Bible passage with your current struggle in mind.

5. Why is God a better refuge than food?

6. What can you thank Him for today?

Emotional Eating
Renewing Questions

1. What's going on in your life right now that's making you want to eat?

2. What emotion are you experiencing?

3. Will eating make you feel better? If so, for how long?

4. Will eating solve your problems?

5. Will eating create any new problems? Explain.

6. What do your boundaries protect you from? Do you need protection today?

7. What do you think God wants to teach you through this trial?

8. Is there anything you need to accept?

9. What can you thank God for in this situation?

Going to God versus Going to Food

Scripture Meditation

*My God will supply all your needs according
to His riches in glory in Christ Jesus.*
Philippians 4:19

1. Often, we eat to satisfy some need in our lives. Think of your current life. What's going on right now that's making you want to break your boundaries?

2. What will happen if you go to food to fill that need?

3. What will happen if you go to God to fill that need?

4. God wants us to go to Him for help with life, but He's also equipped us with resources to solve problems. Can you think of any practical things you could do right now that would be more helpful than eating to satisfy your current need? Brainstorm as many ideas as possible, including renewing your mind about your current struggle.

5. Spend some time visiting with God about your current dilemma. Lean into His comfort, love, and protection, and ask Him for wisdom in how to handle your current situation. Consider doing one of the practical suggestions you made in the last question.

"I Need a Little Excitement in My Life!"

Truth Journaling

Write truths for the following beliefs.

Beliefs

1. I deserve a treat since this is such a boring day.
2. It's too long to wait until the next time I get to eat.
3. I need a little excitement in my life right now.
4. If I don't have a treat, I will go crazy.
5. One little treat won't hurt.

Truths

1.

2.

3.

4.

5.

Reward Eating

Renewing Questions

1. Why do you feel like you deserve a reward?

2. Will you break your boundaries if you reward yourself with food?

   Yes: If so, which boundary will you break? Is that a good boundary? Why or why not?

   No: If not, will you be more likely to break your boundaries later if you reward yourself with food now? Why or why not?

3. Can you think of anything else you could reward yourself with besides food? List a few options.

4. What will happen if you continue to reward yourself with food whenever you accomplish something?

5. Do you want that to happen?

6. When you think of the life you want to live, are boundaries a blessing or a curse?

7. What do boundaries add to your life?

8. What will your life and body look like a couple of months down the road if you develop the habit of consistently following your boundaries?

9. When you think of all you'll gain, is it worth the sacrifice?

When You're Annoyed with Someone

Renewing Questions

1. Why are you annoyed? Be specific.

2. Are you surprised by this person's behavior? Why or why not?

3. Why does their behavior bother you so much? Do you think their behavior bothers God? Why or why not?

4. Do you think this person is open to change? If so, do you think God wants you to talk to them? If not, what will happen if you try to change a person who doesn't want to be changed?

5. How do you think God wants you to respond to this person? What would you need to give up, if anything, to respond the way God wants you to respond?

6. Do you love God (or this person) enough to make that sacrifice?

7. Is there anything you need to accept?

8. What do you think God wants to do for you in the midst of this difficult situation?

9. Do you need to add some boundaries to this relationship? If so, what boundaries could you actually enforce? (If this relationship is abusive or potentially abusive, please get help as soon as possible.)

10. What can you thank God for in this situation? Don't forget to include the things you like about this person.

Perfectionism Eating
Renewing Questions

1. What are you trying to do perfectly?

2. What would perfection look like in this case? (Give a thorough description.)

3. Are you capable of making that happen? (Be realistic.)

4. Are you simply trying to excel (a good thing) or do you feel like you have to be perfect?

5. Why do you feel like you have to be perfect?

6. Does God think you have to be perfect? Why or why not?

7. Is there anything God wants you to do?

8. Is there anything you need to accept?

9. What can you thank God for in this situation?

Turning to Food for Comfort
Scripture Meditation

May our Lord Jesus Christ Himself and God our Father, who has loved us and given us eternal comfort and good hope by grace, comfort and strengthen your hearts in every good work and word.
2 Thessalonians 2:16-17

1. So often we turn to food rather than God for comfort. Describe the whole experience of turning to food for comfort—from the moment the idea pops into your mind to how you feel afterward.

2. Based on your response to the last question, is food a good comforter? Why or why not?

3. In Jeremiah 2:13, the Lord says, "My people have committed two evils: they have forsaken Me, the fountain of living waters, to hew for themselves cisterns, broken cisterns that can hold no water." In what way is comfort eating like trying to fill a leaky cistern?

4. Review today's Bible passage. How is God's comfort different from the comfort we get from food? List as many differences as possible.

5. Spend some time going to God for comfort. Spill out your troubles to Him, then ask Him to help you see your trials from a biblical perspective. Soak in His love and ask Him for strength and wisdom.

Eating After a Vacation

Truth Journaling

Write truths for the following beliefs.

Beliefs

1. I deserve some treats today.
2. After all I just got back from a trip!
3. Life is so dull and boring here.
4. Eating is the one fun thing I can do since the rest of life is so drab.
5. I'll just renew my mind after I eat, and then it will be okay.

Truths

1.

2.

3.

4.

5.

"I'm So Tired!"

Renewing Questions

1. Will this food wake you up for the rest of the day, or will it only wake you up for a short time?

2. What will happen the rest of the day if you break your boundaries now?

3. Is it worth the sacrifice just to be awake for a short time?

4. What is it you need right now?

5. What's the best way to meet that need?

6. What can you be thankful for in this situation?

When You Want Fun, Exciting, and Easy
Scripture Meditation

All discipline for the moment seems not to be joyful, but
sorrowful; yet to those who have been trained by it, afterwards
it yields the peaceful fruit of righteousness.
Hebrews 12:11

1. I'm a big fan of fun, exciting, and easy. So when life is hard or boring, I'm tempted to break my boundaries. What hard or boring thing are you going through right now?

2. What are the benefits of breaking boundaries and eating when life is hard or boring?

3. What are the benefits of facing your problems (including the problem of a boring life) and going to God for help with those problems?

4. The redeeming aspect of problems is that God can use them as discipline in our lives to help us mature. Can you think of any ways God might want you to grow in your character through this current hard or boring situation?

5. In addition to growing in our character, it's also helpful to find practical solutions to our problems. Brainstorm different solutions to your current boring or hard situation and write your ideas below.

6. Spend some time visiting with God about your ideas, then lean into His comfort, strength, and love. Accept what you need to accept and thank God that He is enough no matter what life brings.

The Mom Life

Truth Journaling

Write truths for the following beliefs.

Beliefs

1. I don't want these leftovers to go to waste.
2. I am so overworked that I deserve a treat.
3. Since I always have to be the bad guy and get everyone to do what they don't want to do, the least I can do is have a treat.
4. If the kids are all having a snack, I should have one too.
5. The kids are finally asleep; this is the perfect time for a treat.

Truths

1.

2.

3.

4.

5.

Learning to Be Content

Renewing Questions

1. Why are you unhappy?

2. What do you think will make you happy?

3. Will that really make you happy? Why or why not?

4. Are you able to create the conditions you think will make you happy?

5. Is God enough to satisfy you, even if you don't get what you want? What is one thing you can do to draw closer to Him today?

6. What is one thing you can do to show love to others today? Be specific.

7. Is there anything you need to accept?

8. Is there anything you need to hold with open hands?

9. What can you thank God for in this situation?

"My Life Is a Wreck!"

Truth Journaling

Write truths for the following beliefs.

Beliefs

1. My life is such a wreck!
2. Everything is going wrong.
3. I can't handle it.
4. I need to eat.
5. I deserve this one indulgence since everything in my life is so terrible.

Truths

1.

2.

3.

4.

5.

Relationship Troubles
Option Chart

The headings at the top of this chart show the things we want. The rows on the left show our options. Use up and down arrows and comments to evaluate your real-life options so you can see which option would be best.

Options	To Have This Person Change and Act the Way You Want Them to Act	Peace and Joy	Relationship with God
Ask this person to change, then sit back and be thankful as you watch the person change this instant and be the person you always wanted them to be.	NOT	AN	OPTION!
Keep nagging at them to change—either with direct remarks or subtle little comments.			
End your relationship with them or withdraw from them emotionally and make it a shallow relationship.			

Act all nicey-nice on the outside but continue to resent them on the inside.			
Give them the silent treatment.			
Withhold things they want in the relationship—make them earn your love.			
Talk to a friend or loved one often about how terrible this person is.			
Drown your sorrows in food, alcohol, the internet, etc.			
Forgive them, love them with a 1 Corinthians 13 love, accept their weaknesses, then talk to God and possibly a Christian counselor about what actions to take if any.			

"Of Course I'm Worried!"
Scripture Meditation

The LORD is my light and my salvation; Whom shall I fear? The LORD is the defense of my life; Whom shall I dread? When evildoers came upon me to devour my flesh, My adversaries and my enemies, they stumbled and fell. Though a host encamp against me, My heart will not fear; Though war arises against me, In spite of this I shall be confident. One thing I have asked from the LORD, that I shall seek: That I may dwell in the house of the LORD all the days of my life, to behold the beauty of the LORD and to meditate in His temple.

Psalm 27:1-4

1. What are you afraid of or worried about today?

2. When others tell us not to worry, it's easy to blow them off and say, "Hey, you would worry too if you had my life." Yet David—a man who was often in danger of being killed by his enemies—tells us, "Hey, you don't need to worry." According to his psalm, why do you not need to worry, even if your worry does come true? List as many reasons as possible.

3. Now think about the comfort you get if you go to food for your worries. Review the list of things you wrote in the last question. How does food compare to God?

4. How does the situation you're worried about look from a cultural perspective? How does it look from a biblical perspective?

5. Spend some time visiting with God about your worries, accepting what you need to accept, making a plan to act if you need to act, and shifting your trust to God.

"I Wish I Had My Old Life Back"

Truth Journaling

Write truths for the following beliefs.

1. Life is so terrible now.
2. It will never be good again.
3. There is nothing worth living for now.
4. I should take a break from my boundaries until I get used to this new life.
5. That will make me feel better.

Truths

1.

2.

3.

4.

5.

Boredom Eating
Renewing Questions

1. What do you feel like eating?

2. Will you break a boundary if you eat that?

   Yes: If so, which boundary will you break? Is that a good boundary? Explain.

   No: If not, will you be more likely to break your boundaries later if you eat this? Why or why not?

3. How much time do you need to fill until your next meal or snack?

4. Would eating be a good way to fill this time?

5. What are some other things you could do with this block of time? List a few ideas.

6. What would be the best use of your time right now?

7. What would you gain by using your time this way?

8. Is there anything you need to accept?

"I Have to Be Skinny"

Lies You May Have Learned Growing Up, Part 1

Truth Journaling

Circle any of the lies you learned about your body while growing up—from your family or the culture—and then replace each lie with a truth.

Lies

1. I have to be skinny to be acceptable.

2. Overweight people are ugly.

3. People are talking about me behind my back and saying terrible things about me when I'm overweight.

4. If I want to get (and keep) a spouse, I need to be skinny.

5. If I get too skinny, I'll get unwanted attention.

Truths

1.

2.

3.

4.

5.

Lies You May Have Learned Growing Up, Part 2

Truth Journaling

Circle any of the lies you learned growing up (or through your culture) about your body, then record the truth for each lie.

Lies

1. I need to go on a diet and lose weight before any big event.
2. People won't like me unless I'm skinny (or God won't like me unless I'm skinny).
3. It's incredibly important to be skinny—more important than being kind and loving, for example, or smart and interesting.
4. If I get too skinny, people will think I'm a snob.
5. If I'm overweight, people will think I'm a loser.

Truths

1.

2.

3.

4.

5.

When You Feel Like Others Are Judging You for Your Weight

Scripture Meditation

There is now no condemnation for those who are in Christ Jesus. For the law of the Spirit of life in Christ Jesus has set you free from the law of sin and death.

Romans 8:1-2

1. What just happened that made you (feel like a loser, beat yourself up, etc.)?

2. Do you ever feel like there's an imaginary crowd out there condemning you for being overweight? If so, who do you think would realistically be in that crowd? Is anyone actually condemning you in real life? Name names.

3. It wouldn't surprise me if the crowd were much smaller than you originally thought—and it also wouldn't surprise me if *you* were in that crowd as we're often our own worst critics. How does it affect

your attitude and desire to continue working on breaking free from the control of food when you beat yourself up for breaking your boundaries?

4. While we can't control what others think, we *can* control what we think. How would your attitude and actions change if you were to accept the grace God gives, see yourself through His eyes, and respect others enough to assume they're capable of loving and respecting you even if you're overweight (unless they've told you otherwise)?

5. Spend some time visiting with God about what just happened. Try to see yourself through His eyes, accept the grace He gives, and soak in His all-encompassing love.

"If Only I Were Thin"
Truth Journaling

Write truths for the following beliefs.

Beliefs

1. I'm not thin enough.
2. I need to be skinny to be acceptable.
3. I'm not attractive because I'm fat.
4. If only I were thin, life would be good.
5. Everyone thinks I'm a loser because I'm overweight

Truths

1.

2.

3.

4.

5.

When You Don't Feel Beautiful
Scripture Meditation

How beautiful you are, my darling,
How beautiful you are!
Song of Solomon 4:1

1. Picture God saying those words to you. How does it make you feel?

2. If you can't picture God saying those words to you, there's probably someone in your current or past life who told you that you have to be skinny to be acceptable. How do you think God feels about this Hollywood philosophy that you need to be thin to be acceptable? Why do you think He feels that way?

3. Read 1 Samuel 16:7: "The Lord said to Samuel, "Do not look at his appearance or at the height of his stature, because I have rejected him; for God sees not as man sees, for man looks at the outward appearance, but the Lord looks at the heart." According to that passage, what features does God consider most important when He considers how beautiful a person is?

4. List at least five things that are beautiful about you. Include at least one outside attribute (beautiful eyes, gorgeous hair) and four inside attributes (kind, compassionate, patient, friendly).

5. Spend some time thanking God for the ways He has made you beautiful. Ask Him to help you forget this whole idea that you have to be skinny to be beautiful on the outside and help you instead focus on efforts to be beautiful on the inside.

"This Person Will Reject Me If I Don't Lose Weight"
Scripture Meditation

Since we have so great a cloud of witnesses surrounding us, let us also lay aside every encumbrance and the sin which so easily entangles us, and let us run with endurance the race that is set before us, fixing our eyes on Jesus, the author and perfecter of faith, who for the joy set before Him endured the cross, despising the shame, and has sat down at the right hand of the throne of God.

Hebrews 12:1-2

1. Do you ever feel like you have to be skinny to be happy? If so, what do you think causes you to feel that way?

2. The writer of Hebrews tells us to fix our eyes on Jesus, but so often we instead fix our eyes on all the people who have condemned us for being overweight in the past and all the people who may be condemning us right now. What happens when you focus (either consciously or unconsciously) on people who might condemn you for being overweight?

3. What will happen if you instead focus your eyes on Jesus, the author and perfecter of faith?

4. Can you think of any lies you'll need to "throw off" in order to keep your eyes on Jesus? (For example, one lie you may need to throw off is "I need to make everyone happy.")

5. Spend some time visiting with God and shifting your focus from what others think to what God thinks and how much He loves you. Here are some verses to help: 1 Samuel 16:7; Psalm 139:14; Romans 8:1, 38; Hebrews 4:15-16.

"I'll Never Be Skinny Enough for This Event"

Option Chart

The headings at the top of this chart show the things we want. The rows on the left show our options. Use up and down arrows and comments to evaluate your real-life options so you can see which option would be best.

Options	Peace and Joy, Including Enjoying the Event	Have the People at the Event Accept Me and Like Me	Personal Growth
Go back in time and change how I ate so I don't have to worry about being overweight at this event.	NOT	AN	OPTION!
Don't go to the event. Make an excuse so I don't have to put myself in a place where someone might judge me.			
Go to the event but try to be as inconspicuous as possible so no one notices me. Then leave as early as possible.			

Go to the event but assume that everyone is judging me for how I look. Keep thinking about who might be judging me and let that keep me from enjoying the event.			
Go to the event and enjoy it. Live it up and love peo-ple! Pray through 1 Corinthians 13 before the event so I go into it focused on loving others rather than on how I look.			

After a Bad Weigh-In

Renewing Questions

1. What were you expecting to lose this week?

2. Do you think that was a realistic expectation? Why or why not?

3. Based on your past experiences with weight loss, does your weight usually go down in a nice, neat, always-predictable curve? If not, what usually happens?

4. Is it more important to lose weight or to consistently renew your mind so you change the way you think about food? Explain.

5. On a scale of 1 to 10, how diligent have you been about renewing your mind this week?

6. What would you gain by giving up your hopes for a quick fix to this problem and accepting the fact that this isn't going to be easy?

7. What do you think God wants to teach you through this trial?

8. Is there anything you need to accept?

9. What can you thank God for in this situation?

When You Feel Like You Have to Be Skinny
Option Chart

The headings at the top of this chart show the things we want. The rows on the left show our options. Use up and down arrows and comments to evaluate your real-life options so you can see which option would be best. (Note: You can see how I filled out this chart in Appendix B.)

Options	To Be at a Healthy Weight	Peace and Joy	Relationship with God
To be skinny right now this very instant.	**NOT**	**AN**	**OPTION!**
Look at myself in the mirror and think about how terrible I look.			
Worry about what people think and assume that everyone is judging me for being overweight.			
Think to myself, *Why can't I be as skinny as this person?* whenever I see a beautiful skinny person on social media.			

Spend a lot of time exercising, researching fitness tips and diets, and/or obsessing over what boundaries to use so I can be sure to get this weight off! Do whatever it takes to get it off, including things like purging if necessary.			
Use this as an opportunity to learn to be content in all situations. Embrace life, embrace people, embrace God, and embrace my body in its as-is condition, being thankful for what it does for me. Continue to follow my boundaries but from an already acceptable position.			

When You Feel Like a Weight-Loss Failure
Truth Journaling

Write truths for the following beliefs.

Beliefs

1. I'm a failure because I can't stick to my eating plan.

2. It is terrible to be an overweight person.

3. I am not worthy in the eyes of the world.

4. I have to be skinny or I'm an utter failure.

5. People will like me better if I'm skinny.

Truths

1.

2.

3.

4.

5.

"I'll Never Lose This Weight"

Discouraged About Weight Loss
Scripture Meditation

I am confident of this very thing, that He who began a good work in you will perfect it until the day of Christ Jesus.
Philippians 1:6

1. Do you ever get discouraged about the constant struggle to gain control of food? If so, how does that make you feel when you think of trying again or continuing on after a failure?

2. Why do you think God doesn't heal us in a flash when it comes to struggling with recurring things like eating too much?

3. James 1:2-4 tells us that God uses our trials to help us grow—to be "perfect and complete, lacking in nothing." What do you think God wants you to learn through the trial of continuing to try to break free from the control of food even though it feels impossible?

4. What hope does today's verse give you for carrying on even though it's hard?

5. Think of what it looks like to try to follow your boundaries in your own strength, then think of what it looks like to do it *with* God, relying on Him for help. Which option would be more profitable, and why would it be more profitable?

6. Think of the day ahead. At what time today do you most need to go to God for help with following your boundaries? What could you do with Him to gain that help?

7. Set an alarm on your phone if you'd like to commit to what you suggested in the last question. Spend some time visiting with God about anything that came up in today's lesson, and thank Him for the truth of today's Bible verses.

"I Really Blew It Today"

Truth Journaling

Write truths for the following beliefs.

Beliefs

1. I really blew it today.

2. I have no self-control.

3. I'm doomed to be overweight for the rest of my life.

4. I might as well eat more since I already blew it.

5. I'll just start again tomorrow.

Truths

1.

2.

3.

4.

5.

When You Have a Bad Weigh-In
Option Chart

The headings at the top of this chart show the things we want. The rows on the left show our options. Use up and down arrows and comments to evaluate your real-life options so you can see which option would be best.

Options	Consistently Following Boundaries	Peace and Joy	To Keep God First in My Life, Holding Both Food and "Skinny" with Open Hands
To immediately lose as much weight as I want.	**NOT**	**AN**	**OPTION!**
Go immediately to the bakery and have a large cinnamon roll with frosting because if I'm not going to lose weight anyway, why bother?			
Get totally discouraged and think I will never, *ever* get over this.			

Assume that my boundaries don't work and that's why I didn't lose weight. Immediately start looking for new boundaries and eat as much as I want today since I'll start with new boundaries tomorrow!			
Complain to my friend that all I do is suffer with nothing to show for it even if I'm only suffering from 7:00 a.m. to 5:00 p.m. and breaking my boundaries every night.			
Think back to how I ate last week to see if I could realistically expect to lose weight, remember that it's not uncommon to go a couple weeks without losing weight even if I'm following my boundaries, and renew since I'll be more tempted to break my boundaries than usual.			

Tired of the Struggle
Scripture Meditation

I waited patiently for the LORD;
And He inclined to me and heard my cry.
He brought me up out of the pit of destruction, out of the miry clay,
And He set my feet upon a rock making my footsteps firm.
He put a new song in my mouth, a song of praise to our God;
Many will see and fear
And will trust in the LORD.

Psalm 40:1-3

1. What's going on in your weight-loss journey (or life) that's making you so discouraged?

2. According to today's passage, why can you hope even though this area of your life has been such a struggle? List as many reasons as possible.

3. This passage talks about putting our trust in God. How would you define *trust*?

4. According to your definition, is a specific weight or body size (or whatever else you're seeking) a good thing to put your trust in? Why or why not?

5. What do you think would happen if you were to (a) calmly renew your mind in writing every time you break your boundaries for the next month (b) try to hold both food and "skinny" with open hands, and (c) shift your trust to God?

6. Pray through these verses with your current struggle in mind and try shifting your trust to God as you do so.

Obsessing over Weight Loss

Truth Journaling

Write truths for the following beliefs.

Beliefs

1. I need to find the perfect boundaries.

2. If I don't know (the exact calories in what I'm eating, if I'm truly hungry enough to eat, if they'll have healthy choices at the potluck, etc.), I won't lose weight.

3. I should think about changing my boundaries.

4. I gained half a pound. I am *so* fat!

5. I need to (exercise for two hours, eat only 500 calories tomorrow, etc.) to make up for what I just ate.

Truths

1.

2.

3.

4.

5.

"I Might as Well Eat!"

Renewing Questions

1. Are you one of those rare people who can follow your boundaries effortlessly and perfectly without ever breaking them? If not, what's the sad truth you'll have to accept right from the beginning?

2. Since you can't go back and change what you ate today, what do you think God wants you to do now? Circle one.

   a. Forget about the boundaries the rest of the day and start fresh in the morning.

   b. Beat yourself up.

   c. Remember that you're in a spiritual battle. Continue to fight the battle with spiritual weapons, knowing that you'll fail at times. Be extra diligent with your weapons in the next 24 hours so you don't break your boundaries again.

3. Which option are you inclined to take? Why?

4. What are the odds you could take that option without regretting it later?

5. If you want to live a life with boundaries, will you have to stop breaking them at some point?

6. What would be the advantage of stopping today?

7. What will your life and body look like a few months down the road if you develop the habit of consistently following your boundaries?

8. When you think of what you'll gain, is it worth the sacrifice to follow your boundaries the rest of the day?

When You Are Sick to Death of Your Boundaries
Scripture Meditation

*We also exult in our tribulations, knowing that tribulation brings about
perseverance; and perseverance, proven character; and proven character, hope.*
Romans 5:3-4

1. Do you feel like you're suffering when you make yourself try to follow
   your boundaries? Why or why not?

2. Paul tells us to rejoice when we're suffering, and he lists some reasons we
   can rejoice. According to this passage, why can you rejoice when you
   follow your boundaries and give up all those fun eating opportunities?

3. From an eating perspective, the endurance of following our
   boundaries even when we don't want to produces the character trait
   of self-control, which leads to the hope that we can actually break
   free from the control of food. How does focusing on the benefits of
   following your boundaries change your attitude toward boundaries?

4. What can you be thankful for as you continue your pursuit of a lifestyle that includes lifelong boundaries with food? Try to list at least five things.

5. Spend some time thanking God for His goodness as He helps you with this battle to break from the control of food. Ask Him to strengthen you today to follow your boundaries.

"I'll Never Get Over This!"

Truth Journaling

Write truths for the following beliefs.

Beliefs

1. I will gain back my weight.

2. I'll keep going and gain a bunch.

3. I can't control my eating.

4. I can't lose weight and keep it off.

5. I have no willpower.

These beliefs are from one of my own journal entries, dated three months *before* I published my first book, *Freedom from Emotional Eating*. The sixth belief I recorded in my journal was: *How will I be able to sell my book if it doesn't work in my own life?* But here's the truth: It did work! I just kept renewing whenever I broke my boundaries, and I've kept the weight off for 16 years now. You can do it too. Just keep renewing even when you feel like it won't work, and one day you'll look back like I'm doing right now and say, "It worked."

Truths

1.

2.

3.

4.

5.

Regret After Breaking a Major Boundary

Renewing Questions

1. What do you wish you would have done or not done?

2. Do you think God wishes you had done things differently? Why or why not?

3. Since you can't go back and change what you did or didn't do, how do you think God wants you to respond now?

4. How would Satan like you to respond?

5. What can you gain from this experience if you respond the way God wants you to respond?

6. Can God redeem this situation even if you really messed up? Explain.

7. Is there anything you need to accept?

8. Is there anything you need to confess?

9. Do you need to apologize to anyone or make restitution?

10. What can you thank God for in this situation?

When You Feel Like Giving Up
Scripture Meditation

Let us not lose heart in doing good, for in due time we will reap if we do not become weary. So then, while we have opportunity, let us do good to all people, and especially those who are of the household of the faith.

Galatians 6:9-10

1. What happened that made you feel discouraged about your weight-loss journey?

2. Do you think it's possible to go from being controlled by food to being free from the control of food without experiencing days like today? Why or why not?

3. Today's Bible passage tells us to not lose heart in doing good. If you were to do good to yourself in this situation, would you (a) give up on trying to follow your boundaries and go back to an eat-what-you-want-when-you-want lifestyle, (b) beat yourself up and say, "You will never lose this weight, you undisciplined oaf!," or (c) renew your mind and press on with your boundaries even though it's super hard?

Also, what would you advise your loved one to do in this situation? Why would you advise that?

4. According to today's Bible verse, what will happen if you keep "doing good"? What would that look like in your life?

5. Spend some time visiting with God about whatever happened to discourage you today. Ask Him to give you hope and strength to carry on, then thank Him for all the good He has already done in your life through this weight-loss journey.

Eating After a Weigh-In or Big Event
Truth Journaling

Write truths for the following beliefs.

Beliefs

1. There's no need to be skinny since this is over.
2. I should live it up after all that suffering.
3. I deserve it after all that sacrificing to get to a lower weight.
4. I can eat now without consequences.
5. This will be the good life!

Truths

1.

2.

3.

4.

5.

"This Isn't Going as Well as I Thought It Would"

Renewing Questions

1. What were you expecting to gain, accomplish, or achieve?

2. What happened instead?

3. Based on your past experiences with weight loss, does success usually come in a nice, neat, always-moving-upward curve? If not, how does it usually come?

4. Do you think this is just a minor setback, or is it the death of your goal to be free from the control of food? Explain.

5. What will you need to do if you want to be successful with breaking free from the control of food?

6. What do you think God wants to teach you through this trial?

7. Is there anything you need to accept?

8. Is there anything you need to trust God with?

9. What can you thank God for in this situation?

When You're Beating Yourself Up About What You Just Ate

Scripture Meditation

Straightening up, Jesus said to her, "Woman, where are they? Did no one condemn you?" She said, "No one, Lord." And Jesus said, "I do not condemn you, either. Go. From now on sin no more."

John 8:10-11

1. What just happened that made you start beating yourself up?

2. Why do you suppose Jesus didn't condemn the woman who committed adultery in today's Bible passage, even though you could make the argument that she also didn't have any willpower?

3. Romans 2:4 tells us that God's kindness leads us to repentance. What's the difference between repentance and self-condemnation? Which one would be more helpful and why?

4. When we beat ourselves up, it keeps us from going to God for help and learning from the experience. Think about your last overeating session. What fueled the desire to overeat? Can you think of anything you could do on a practical or spiritual level to help the next time this situation crops up?

5. Spend some time visiting with Jesus about what just happened, repenting if necessary, and asking Him—the One Hebrews 4:15-16 tells us was tempted in the same way you are tempted—to help you see life, food, and yourself as He sees you.

"I Should Be Losing More Than This!"

Truth Journaling

Write truths for the following beliefs.

Beliefs

1. I've been good for [amount of time], and I'm not losing anything. (Note: When you write your belief, be honest about whether you've really been keeping to your boundaries.)

2. I deserve to lose more after all that suffering!

3. This isn't worth it if I'm not losing weight.

4. I should just give up.

5. I'll never get over this.

Truths

1.

2.

3.

4.

5.

When You Don't Feel Like Renewing
Advantages-and-Disadvantages Chart

In the chart below, list the advantages and disadvantages of renewing your mind every time you break (or feel like breaking) your boundaries.

Advantages of Renewing Your Mind	Disadvantages of Renewing Your Mind

1. After looking at both columns, is it worth taking the time to renew your mind? Why or why not?

2. What could keep you from renewing?

3. How could you overcome that obstacle?

4. Are there any action steps you'd like to take based on what you learned today?

"Life Will Be Terrible If I Don't Lose Weight!"

Renewing Questions

1. What is your goal?

2. What will you need to do to accomplish your goal? Be specific.

3. How would you define success with this goal?

4. Is it a given that if you do what you need to do, you'll be successful? Why or why not?

5. How do you think God would define success with this project?

6. Is His definition of success easier to achieve than yours? Why or why not?

7. What would be the advantage of going to God for help with this goal, including going to Him for help to see the project through His eyes?

8. Which would be a better reward: (1) intense fellowship with God as you go to Him for help and keep Him (rather than the goal) first in your life, or (2) achieving your weight-loss goal? What sacrifices will you have to make to get the better reward?

9. Are God's lessons and love in the midst of a trial a reward in and of themselves?

10. What can you thank God for in this situation?

After a Bad Night of Eating

Option Chart

The headings at the top of this chart show the things we want. The rows on the left show our options. Use up and down arrows and comments to evaluate your real-life options so you can see which option would be best.

Options	Consistently Following Boundaries	Peace and Joy	Maturity
To not have binged (or broken your boundaries)	**NOT**	**AN**	**OPTION!**
Go into self-condemnation mode. Say things like, "How could I have so little self-control?" or "I should be over this by now!"			
Take it easy for a few days—try to follow my boundaries, but if I can't, it's not a big deal since I seem to be in boundary-breaking mode.			

Try super hard to follow my boundaries the rest of the week but don't take the time to renew my mind.			
Recognize that sometimes I'll break my boundaries (these things happen), and continue trying to follow my boundaries. Renew my mind as much as possible the next few days so I'll have the best possible chance of actually being able to follow them.			

"This Is Too Hard!"
Scripture Meditation

He disciplines us for our good, so that we may share His holiness. All discipline for the moment seems not to be joyful, but sorrowful; yet to those who have been trained by it, afterwards it yields the peaceful fruit of righteousness.
Hebrews 12:10-11

1. The writer of Hebrews mentions that all discipline is sorrowful in the moment. Do you ever feel like it's painful to follow your boundaries? If so, what makes it painful?

2. Not only is it painful to follow our boundaries, but it can also be painful to renew our minds about eating. Do you ever feel like it's painful to do one of these renewing exercises before or after you break your boundaries? If so, what makes it painful?

3. It's interesting that we would *expect* pain if we were to train for a marathon, but we often think following our boundaries should be easy—that we shouldn't have to put any time and effort into renewing

our minds so we can be transformed. Why do you suppose we think
that way?

4. The writer of Hebrews says we'll experience the peaceful fruit of
   righteousness if we allow ourselves to be trained by the discipline.
   Think of the life of eating what you want when you want versus a life
   of following your boundaries perfectly, even on the days it's painful.
   Which life would be more peaceful one day into the discipline? Which
   life would be more peaceful three months into the discipline? Explain.

5. Spend some time visiting with God about the life He wants for you,
   which I'm guessing may also be the life you want for you. Ask Him for
   strength to follow through on your discipline today. Also remember
   that the peaceful fruit of righteousness comes *after* the discipline. It's
   not very peaceful while the battle is raging.

After a Binge

Truth Journaling

Write truths for the following beliefs.

Beliefs

1. I might as well have more since I already broke my boundaries.

2. One more won't hurt.

3. After all, I already broke my boundaries—I should live it up!

4. I'm such a failure.

5. I'll never get over this.

Truths

1.

2.

3.

4.

5.

Lifelong Boundaries
Advantages-and-Disadvantages Chart

One way to renew our minds is to think of the benefits and consequences of our actions. In the chart below, describe each life as fully as possible. For example, one of the characteristics of a life of consistently following eating boundaries is that you wake up each day without regret about what you ate the night before. Another characteristic is that you can maintain a healthy weight. A characteristic of the eating-what-I-want-when-I-want life is that you may struggle with diabetes one day or other health consequences. Another characteristic is that your clothes won't fit.

A Life of Consistently Following Eating Boundaries	A Life of Eating What I Want When I Want

1. After looking at both columns, which life would you rather live—a life of no boundaries, lifelong boundaries and following them, or lifelong boundaries and only following them when you feel like following them?

2. What will you gain if you live a life of having lifelong boundaries and consistently following them every day, every hour, even when you don't feel like it?

3. What will you have to accept if you choose that life?

Appendix A

"I Don't Want to Renew My Mind"

Following is an example of how you could fill out the chart "I Don't Want to Renew My Mind" on page 90.

Options	Peace and Joy	Closeness to God	Consistently Following Boundaries
To be able to lose weight and keep it off without having to renew my mind.	**NOT**	**AN**	**OPTION!** (Romans 12:2)
Give up on renewing and just try to follow my weight-loss plan.	↓ I can't do this in my own strength, and failure is stressful and depressing!	↓ I won't be going to God for help, so I won't grow closer to Him.	↓ I need to renew if I want to have the strength to follow my boundaries.
Renew when it's convenient, but don't renew when it's not convenient—when I'm on a trip for example, or there are a lot of people in my house, or when I'm working outside the home.	↓ These are the times I'm most likely to break boundaries, so I'd better find a way to renew.	↓ This this won't affect my relationship with God that much, but it would be a good way to connect during these times when I have a hard time connecting with Him.	↓ Again, I need to learn to follow my boundaries in these situations, so I need to make the sacrifice to renew when I'm in these situations.
Renew once in the morning, but then don't renew again the rest of the day, even if I break my boundaries.	↓ This won't do the trick as I won't be doing battle against the lies that make me eat. Generals don't win battles by only fighting in the morning!	↓ The more I go to God for help throughout the day, the closer I'll feel to Him.	↓ I need to renew in the moment of temptation to have the strength and desire to follow my boundaries—and these moments of temptation usually occur later in the day.

Renew my mind but don't put my whole effort into it. Just write enough to check it off my list, but not enough to change the way I think.	↓ This will make me even more stressed out and depressed because I'll think, *I'm going to all this effort, and it's not working!* When really I'm only doing a half-hearted effort.	↓ Just as I want the people close to me to put effort into changing the things they need to change, God wants me to put effort into changing the things *He* wants me to change! And although He'll love me regardless, renewing will make *me* feel closer to Him.	↓ Again, this won't change me and I won't experience the benefits of the boundaries lifestyle if I don't renew, since I can't gain that lifestyle in my own strength.
Recognize that discipline is not fun in the moment, but afterward, I will reap joy (Hebrews 12:11). Renew my mind every single time I break my boundaries, even if I'm sick to death of it!	↑↓ This is my best chance for peace and joy as it is my best chance of breaking free from the control of food. Will it be more stressful in the moment? Yes—it's far easier to eat than it is to allow God to search me and know my thoughts. But each time I renew, I'll feel that peace and joy that comes from seeing life from a biblical perspective. (Note: If you're not feeling peace and joy most of the time after renewing, read chapters 5–7 to see if you need to follow any of the renewing tips in those chapters.)	↑ When I take the time to renew, I'm learning to look at life from God's perspective. This will make me feel closer to Him.	↑ This is my best chance of experiencing the benefits because it is my best chance of breaking free from the control of food and learning to follow and even embrace and enjoy my boundaries.

Appendix B

When You Feel Like You Have to Be Skinny

Following is an example of how you could fill out the chart "When You Feel Like You Have to Be Skinny" on page 218.

Options	To Be at a Healthy Weight	Peace and Joy	Relationship with God
To be skinny right now this very instant.	**NOT**	**AN**	**OPTION!**
Look at myself in the mirror and think about how terrible I look.	↓ This just sends me into Despair Land and makes me want to eat. Surprisingly, I'll have a *better* chance of losing weight if I learn to accept my body in its as-is condition.	↓ This just stresses me out because I feel like I have to be perfect. The Bible says I can learn to be content in *all* situations. That would include this situation—with my as-is body!	↓ God wants me to be thankful and dwell on the good. When I condemn my body, I'm not being thankful! Instead, I'm being demanding and saying, "I have to have the perfect body to be happy!" This draws me away from God.
Worry about what people think and assume that everyone is judging me for being overweight.	↓ Again, this makes me overeat! Which makes me gain weight.	↓ When I do this, not only do I get depressed, I also isolate, and this makes me miss out on the joy of relationships. Most people couldn't care less how much I weigh. I need to remember that!	↓ God wants me to think the best of people. I'm not doing that when I assume they're judging me. Also, even if they are judging me, God doesn't want me to seek the approval of people but to instead walk in the safety and confidence of His love and how *He* sees me!

Think to myself, *Why can't I be as skinny as this person?* whenever I see a beautiful skinny person on social media.	↓ This just makes me want to eat because life seems so unfair. And that will make me gain weight.	↓ This is a recipe for comparison and depression—not peace and joy!	↓ The Bible tells me not to envy or be jealous. Instead of being grateful for a body that works and *moves*, I'm ungrateful because it's not perfect! This draws me away from God. I should probably think about spending less time on social media.
Spend a lot of time exercising, researching fitness tips and diets, and/or obsessing over what boundaries to choose so I can be sure to get this weight off! Do whatever it takes to get it off, including things like purging.	↑↓ This could possibly help me lose weight, but that weight loss would come at the expense of my health and other things that are more important, not to mention the fact that I could be tempted to lose down to an unhealthy low weight.	↓ Obsession does not lead to peace and joy! Instead I'll always be stressed, wondering if I'm doing enough to lose or maintain my weight. Also, if I feel like I have to be skinny to be acceptable, I'll never be skinny enough to satisfy me. I can always get a little fitter or a little skinnier.	↓ God doesn't want me to make an idol of skinny. When I focus all my attention on getting or maintaining skinny, I don't feel close to God. The more I let go and hold skinny with open hands, the closer I'll feel to Him.

Use this as an opportunity to learn to be content in all situations. Embrace life, embrace people, embrace God, and embrace my body in its as-is condition, being thankful for what it does for me. Continue to follow my boundaries but from an already acceptable position.	↑ This actually may be my best chance to live at a healthy weight as it will eliminate the portion of emotional eating that I do because I feel like I'll never be able to lose weight and that I *have* to lose it to be acceptable. Those are the feelings that are fueling most of my late-night binge sessions.	↑ This is my best chance for peace and joy since I'm not relying on a number on the scale to be happy and not feeling like, "Oh no, I better lose this weight or it will be terrible!"	↑ This is also my best chance to be close to God since I'm working toward putting Him first in my life and remembering that He is enough—I don't need to be skinny to be happy! It's also my best chance to be close to God because I'll be more likely to go to Him, not diet articles, exercise, healthy eating, etc. for help with life.

About the Author

BARB RAVELING specializes in lies and truth. She has been truth journaling for 20 years and helping others discover lies and truth through her practical Bible studies and books.

Barb is a certified executive Christian coach through Coach Approach Ministries and has extensive postcollege training in both biblical counseling and life coaching. Barb has used her training to help Christians grow through online classes, local workshops and Bible studies, one-on-one coaching, a blog, and two podcasts on Christian growth, *Taste for Truth* and *Christian Habits*. She blogs and podcasts at BarbRaveling.com.

Other Books by Barb Raveling:

Freedom from Emotional Eating

I Deserve a Donut (and Other Lies That Make You Eat)

Taste for Truth

A Renewing of the Mind Project

Rally: A Personal Growth Bible Study

Freedom from Procrastination

James

To learn more about Harvest House books and
to read sample chapters, visit our website:

www.HarvestHousePublishers.com

HARVEST HOUSE PUBLISHERS
EUGENE, OREGON